Live Long,
Die Fast

Live Long, Die Fast

Playing
the Aging Game
to Win

John H. Bland, M.D.

Fairview Press
Minneapolis

Published by Fairview Press, 2450 Riverside Avenue South, Minneapolis, MN 55454.

Library of Congress Cataloging-in-Publication Data

Bland, John H. (John Hardesty), 1917–
Live long, die fast : playing the aging game to win / John H. Bland, M.D.
      p.   cm.
   ISBN 1-57749-012-6 (pbk. : alk. paper)
   1. Aging.   2. Aged—Health and hygiene.   I. Title.
   RA777.6.B58   1997
   613' . 0438—DC20   96–9430
                                  CIP

First Printing: January 1997

Printed in the United States of America
01 00 99 98 97   7 6 5 4 3 2

Cover design: Richard Rossiter

Publisher's Note: Fairview Press publishes books and other materials related to the subjects of social and family issues. Its publications, including *Live Long, Die Fast,* do not necessarily reflect the philosophy of Fairview Hospital and Healthcare Services or their treatment programs.

For a free current catalog of Fairview Press titles, please call this toll-free number: 1-800-544-8207.

TABLE OF CONTENTS

Dedication

Dedicated to my children and grandchildren: John*, Perry, Beth, Linda; Kristin, Mitch, Brooke, Jessica, Melissa, and Kyler. May their lives be long, happy, productive, and full to brimming over.

*He did live fast, happily, and abundantly, if not long.

Acknowledgments

A book like this requires work, aid, and support by many people.

First, Linda Mendenhall Bland, my daughter, my agent, my editor, clearly one of my very best friends. My gratitude for converting a raw manuscript to the finished product, lean, clean, attractive, exciting English prose; for sage guidance in the sale of the manuscript—with tolerance, patience, and superb humor.

To Libits, my wife, for guidance, for support, for belief in the project over thirty years of collecting the data reflected in the finished product; for continuing advice and assessment of appropriateness and comprehensibility of large sections of the text; for the wonderful fun we had in the process.

To Linda Poppe, my respect, gratitude, and admiration for supplying important reprints, suggestions, and clippings on the subject of aging; for typing and retyping the manuscript, converting reams of handwritten, dictated, and extensively edited material; for her workmanship, encouragement, outspoken nature, and skill at correcting errors; for her wit and warm humor, a dear friend of many years. She is happily compulsive, driven to excel, completing a large volume of work quickly while offering compassionate criticism and advice.

To Marie M. McGarry for her library skills and bibliographic references; for her always prompt delivery, doing three days work in one with accuracy and precision. Her vivacity and rapid completion of requests made a contribution to the finished project.

To Cynthia McIlwain Taeuber of the U.S. Department of Commerce, Economics, and Statistics Administration, Bureau of the Census, for her wonderfully complete and highly systematically arranged book, *Sixty-five Plus in America*. The concentrated arrangement of reams of data has allowed me far more comprehension and understanding of all aspects of the United States population over sixty-five years of age.

To Robert N. Butler, the first director of the National Institutes of Aging for the most important book of the hundreds I have read, *Why Survive? Being Old in America*, a Pulitzer Prize winner published in 1975 by Harper Torch Books. Rare it is that a Pulitzer Prize is won for a book on the subject of aging, sociology, science, demographics, government, religion, and politics. I did not just read the book, I studied it page by page.

To James F. Fries, who with Lawrence M. Crapo wrote the book *Vitality and Aging* published in 1981. This book was among the first dealing with the detailed demographics of aging, and contributing pertinent, fresh knowledge on life span and life expectancy.

To Leonard Hayflick, for his many published scientific papers, his discovery that human cells (fibroblasts) have a limited number of divisions (+/- 50), one of the most basic and important contributions to the subject of aging. Hayflick's book *How and Why We Age* (Ballantine Books, 1994) makes a major contribution toward finding the answer to how and why we age, unearthing many critical biological clues.

Preface

No Star in the East

I always knew I was going to die, I just didn't know when. For a while, like my adolescent peers, I was convinced of my own immortality—and acted accordingly. I did not consider death a possibility; death happened to other people. I've given that up now. The evidence is overwhelming—and my mother remembers no star in the east on November 7, 1917, when I was born.

Immortality ruled out as an option, I contemplate my mortality with great interest and enthusiasm. As I researched this book, a simple truth offered comforting relief: There's no such thing as dying of old age. If there's one thing that rivals death on my personal fear scale, it's the conventional specter of "old age." What we most fear is developing a disease that won't kill, but disable us physically and intellectually—leaving us unable to work, feeling sick all the time, depressed, surly, unloving, and unlovable—and still we live on. This specter of decrepitude, to live with no awareness of family, friends, or the environment, is our worst nightmare. Such an end is not a necessary evil—it can be prevented by using all we know about aging.

The stereotype of the aging person is ensconced in the American psyche; most of it is based on folklore and nonsense.

The best remedy for these misconceptions is facts. Here are fourteen of the most common stereotypes of aging, what the majority of people believe. Each fallacy is accompanied by facts, disproving every feature of aging we have feared:

1. Physical aging is a natural process that is unalterable.

On the contrary, studies show that great strides can be made in regaining strength, agility, balance, and independence if a person of any age pursues a regular exercise program. No one is too old to respond to training: Recently ten frail, institutionalized volunteers, age ninety and over, undertook eight weeks of high-intensity resistance training. Strength measurements gained an average of 174 percent among all ten people.

2. The biggest hardship the elderly endure is physical.

The physical changes they experience are trifling compared to their most difficult hurdles: social, political, and employment discrimination. Old age exists only in societies that create it by how they classify people. It could be abolished tomorrow by declassifying and de-stereotyping.

3. Most old people end up living in institutions, nursing homes, hospitals, retirement homes.

The actual figure in the United States among those over 65 years of age is 4 percent.

4. After age sixty-five, it's all downhill.

In reality, 51 percent rate their health as good; 33 percent as fair; and less than 16 percent as poor. Two-thirds of this last group's decline is due to inactivity, boredom, and expectation that infirmity is coming, even inevitable. Over a research period of three to thirteen years, 44 to 58 percent of those over sixty-five returned for check-ups with no detectable deterioration in physical condition—some improved! This is not to say some don't get sick and decline, but when this happens earlier in life it's called illness, not aging.

5. Everyone knows that people over age sixty-five are long past having sex.

We have learned that they are either having sex happily or would welcome the opportunity to have it because they are fully able to enjoy it.

6. Older people are ashamed of their wrinkles and overall appearance.

The unexpected truth is that 66 percent of those over sixty-five like how they look. Even more surprising is that they like the way they look more than any other age group asked! Those over sixty-five tend to be more comfortable with who they are, and less concerned with what others think of them.

7. Old people are alone and lonely, abandoned by family and friends.

Statistics say 80 percent of those over sixty-five live with someone else; 75 percent say they are not often alone; 86 percent saw one or more relatives during the previous week. The same study charted proximity of the nearest child to each person: 28 percent live in the same house; 33 percent live within a ten-minute drive; 23 percent live within an hour of their nearest child. Another fact rarely considered is that you can be alone and not be lonely. You may not need anyone—many older people love being alone. Loneliness is being alone when you don't want to be. This does not mean that none of these people are lonely or neglected. It does mean the stereotyping is way off.

8. Old people are poor and unable to support themselves.

Over the past two decades, the poverty rate of those over sixty-five has dropped from 35 percent to 12 percent. Financial dependency in the United States today is unrelated to how old you are. Fifty percent of American millionaires are over age sixty-five. Your financial future is looking better already!

9. All older people should retire because they can't do a good job.

Older workers have a better attendance record than younger workers. They have fewer disabling and non-disabling injuries, and a lower frequency of accidents. Here is a list of people who have done excellent work late in life: Grandma Moses became a painter at seventy-six and finished her last canvas shortly before her death at one hundred one; Charles de Gaulle left office at age seventy-eight, Churchill at eighty, United States Senator Frances Green at ninety-three; pianist Arthur Rubenstein, born in 1886, gave concerts until recently; George Bernard Shaw was ninety-four when one of his plays was first produced; Golda Meir was seventy-one when she became Prime Minister of Israel.

10. Most old people are constantly in bed with severe illness. They get fractures easily and suffer a slow death.

In truth, those over sixty-five get fewer illnesses than younger people: 1.3 per year as opposed to 2.1 percent for those under age sixty-five. It is true that 81 percent of older people have some chronic problem; but this is not much more than the 54 percent of all people under age sixty-five. Their chronic "problem" may be no more than slight hearing or vision compromise, both of which are correctable.

11. After age sixty-five, your mind will deteriorate and you will eventually become senile.

This is a self-fulfilling prophecy that is almost totally unnecessary. All that really happens is a slight drop in speed of response. Normally, there is no change in intelligence and very little change in memory, and even this can be easily accommodated. Any lessening of acuity that occurs (in the absence of disease) commonly results from boredom, not enough to do, just as a child gets bored without enough to do. These people are often put down by others, and become exasperated. By far the best way to prevent loss of memory or any other mental performance is by continued vigorous and enthusiastic use: ongoing learning, thinking, problem solving, enriching of your environment.

12. As you age, you lose the pleasure in life: your appetite, libido, the ability to sleep well, and a sense of well-being.

On the contrary, a full one-third of those over sixty-five report their best years ever or that they expect the best is yet to come. The problems mentioned have nothing to do with age, they are symptoms of depression. Nowadays most depression can be relieved with exercise and medication. Depression is a biochemical disorder, which is treated as such in younger people, but sadly considered "normal" for aging. The most common cause of suicide in all ages is depression aggravated by sickness or social abuse by society, both things you endure more and more as you age. And you need not!

13. The disengagement from society at age sixty-five is a natural acceptance of old age's limitation, and older people welcome it.

This is how society justifies easing out people it wants to treat as disposable. Those who can make a buck off the elderly will tell you, "People like being kicked out of the living community, put out to pasture so they can finally relax." This smoothing of our guilt is done because if these "inmates" made waves about it, it would be inconvenient for society's planning. This whitewash is ludicrous. Wasting 25 percent of the population doesn't seem to be in anyone's best interest—especially since every one of us eventually join the 25percent.

14. Some health problems and diseases are inevitable; if you live long enough you are bound to get them: arteriosclerosis, arthritis, vision impairment, hearing loss.

Arteriosclerosis is preventable through exercise and nutrition. Besides this, entire societies (Chinese and Japanese) have none. Arthritis in your joints will occur eventually, but it can usually be managed so that it is without symptoms. Though people of all nationalities get osteoarthritis, less than 10 percent of individuals suffer any symptoms at all. Vision and hearing abilities do diminish but both are entirely correctable, and neither are debilitating.

I take pleasure in refuting false beliefs embedded in the American psyche because these convictions block methods of dealing effectively with aging, health, and death. Most younger people believe this, and it becomes a source of anxiety as they grow older. We expect to suffer these changes. How did we get in this mess? There is a steady drip of misinformation that prepares people to be victimized at age sixty-five; the rest of us victimize them until we get there ourselves.

No one enjoys contemplating their own death, but death is a fact of life. The question "would you rather talk about sex or dying?" always draws a unanimous response. And yet seriously planning, considering death's inevitability, makes a lot of sense. No one wants to die slowly—over a period of years—that's what we fear most.

It has become clear over the last fifty years that we are living longer. It is also evident that our life span and maximum life potential are programmed in our genes. Diseases and trauma superimpose themselves over our genetic programming, compromising physical and sometimes intellectual function. These environmental villains (disease and trauma) shorten life and slow the process of death. In our hearts and souls, we all really want to live long, to our absolute maximum duration—and then die in seconds, minutes, or hours (at the most days or weeks, certainly not months or years).

Like every unknown we encounter in life, the more we learn about aging and death, the more relaxed and confident we can feel about it. There are but two things I'm absolutely certain about every second: (1) I shall be dead some day; and (2) I'm not dead now. My goal is to extend, for as long as I can, the time between now and my death, to die young as late as possible. To live long and die fast...in good health! Solidly based scientific and demographic observations of the past fifty years support the feasibility of this goal. The diseases and trauma we die of are largely preventable—or, at least, postponable. Furthermore, most of them are beyond the reach of doctors to prevent, for they are governed by life style: attitudes, education, diet, environment, exercise—all of which you can influence and modify. The next great breakthrough in medicine and health will be to fend for yourself. Do all that you can, beginning as early as you can—even as a teenager—to live a life plan designed to realize your maximum genetic endowment. Take full advantage of the genes of your species—Homo sapiens. You have a pre-ordained life span and maximum life potential. Take charge of it! Only recently have we noticed that more of us are realizing only about five-sixths of our maximum life potential. For the past decade, the fastest growing segment of the United States population was those over eighty-five years. But that is now old news. According to the U.S. Census Bureau, the current, fastest growing segment of the population is those over one hundred years of age. Let's latch onto all our potential.

A consensus among researchers on human aging declared that a reasonable assessment of our species potential for longevity is around 120 years—and we know for sure that one member of our species is living today at 121 years. Genesis 6:3 says "My spirit cannot be indefinitely responsible for human beings, who are only flesh; let the time allowed be a hundred and twenty years." —New Jerusalem Bible translation. (I guess the Lord knew all along.) Too few of us are living long and dying fast, and remaining functional and independent up to death. The unproclaimed secret is that it is an achievable goal. People should adopt the lifestyle, attitude, and practices leading to a long life in their twenties and thirties, though it is never too late to begin. A highly favorable response to the whole program presented here will occur at any age.

When I embarked on this book, I expected consolation. Like everyone, fear was my predominant emotion connected with death. Who wants to die? Death is not perceived as a pleasant event. What a revitalizing research marathon it has been! I'm now fascinated by my own and everyone else's process of dying. After exhaustive research, in pursuit of absolute truths about aging and death, I have once again recognized that most of this I learned at my mother's knee. I intend my death to be a celebration of a long life. I refuse to leak out of this world—and I think I can pull it off!

Its scope comes as a surprise to me. The aging game is an expanding game, expanding my life when I expected it to diminish. It demands an excellence that I thought (perhaps hoped) would no longer be needed. It begins with an awareness of the pressing need to grow and expand in every sphere of existence. I have no trouble now looking truth in the eye. Honesty is not just the best policy, it is the only policy. Lies and deception are time-consuming...and time is essential.

I now like who I am; I even like the way I look! I am going into extra innings and expecting double plays rather than triple bypasses. Life is a play with a badly written third act—let's rewrite it. Don't let it be all bingo and shuffleboard. My latest goal is to be on the cover of *Seventeen* when I'm eighty-seven, America's oldest living teenager, a geriatric jock! Now in my eightieth year, I regard myself as middle-aged.

This book is about strategies you can start today to assure reaching your deserved life span. Live long, die fast—a laudable goal. Take the first step toward "taking charge." You're only old once! Growing old is too often regarded as an endgame, life winding down in a series of spiraling, smaller moves. As I age, I find that this metaphor does not hold at all. It is not a defensive struggle of ever-more restrictive options. To my surprise and joy, it is a game of verve, imagination, and excitement, filled with opportunity, not a matter of continually seeking greater and greater inner strength. Strength remains, but it is now a matter of faith, courage, hope, and wisdom. Aging is like a sport with childhood, youth, and maturity composing the preparation, training, and conditioning for this great aging game.

Introduction

Don't Act Your Age

Take it easy. Slow down. Let me get that for you. Don't excite yourself. You can't eat those anymore. Relax, let someone else worry about it. You're too old for this. You're too old for that, too. Don't try to do that, you'll hurt yourself. Act your age.

If all this evokes a rank defiance from you, if something within you sees the absence of logic in all this bossing—congratulations! You've taken the first step toward living long and dying fast.

What is "acting your age," anyway? When you are little, it means to behave with more maturity, to quit being silly. When you turn thirty-five, however, society defines "acting your age" as reducing your activity, both mentally and physically. After forty or fifty, "acting your age" implies eliminating most of your physical "play" and diminishing all intellectual expectations simply because "you're not as sharp as you once were."

As I entered my sixth and seventh decades, I vehemently rejected all suggestions to act my age. At the same time, I began collecting evidence to buttress my own personal revolt against stereotypical aging. To my surprise and delight, corroboration for my revolt—both personal and factual—abounded.

1

Live Long, Die Fast

Take your genes, for instance. Your doctor, friends, and family may be urging you to slow down, but if your genes could talk (and who knows more about you), they'd be telling you to get out and run, or at least walk a little, every day. For 40,000 years, the day-to-day life of Homo sapiens was dominated by continuous physical activity, primarily hunting and foraging for food. When survival was at stake, we didn't stand around deciding how or when we were going to fit a workout into our day. Though the advent of agriculture marked the beginning of the end of an extremely active lifestyle, our genes still retain the capacity for fitness. As a result, our overall health still depends on some form of daily movement. We are animals, custom-designed to move most of the time we are awake. Defying the instructions of our genes is tempting fate.

Another surprising contradiction to stereotypical notions about aging has to do with nutrition. Remember being pressed to eat more as a child?

"Be a member of the 'Clean Plate Club.'"

"Think of all the starving children."

"No dessert until you finish your spinach and broccoli."

Such advice, however well-intentioned, has created life-shortening habits and attitudes. Walk down any busy American main street and you'll be struck (perhaps literally) by our collective obesity. Most overweight people are not thinking about their life expectancy and how they have shortened and are continuing to shorten it. The only sure method to increase life expectancy is dietary restriction. Investigators have found that laboratory rats fed a low-calorie diet lived longer than those consuming food at will. "The thin rat goes to the fat rat's funeral." These findings have been repeated in many species, both vertebrate and invertebrate, including pigs, mice, flies, and fish. Dietary restriction preserves the body and promotes longevity, and caloric restriction alters the rate of physiologic decline in animals, postponing the onset of fatal diseases. If, by slowing

2

the rate of senescence, you postpone all physiologic mechanisms of aging, youth could be prolonged and disability compressed into only a very short period before death—hours or even minutes. The data suggest strongly that if Americans from twenty to fifty change their lifestyles, they will prolong their life expectancy.

I found more good news not being publicly reported. Even if you eat all day and don't exercise, your chances of living longer are still better than ever before. An unprecedented phenomenon is taking place: life expectancy for our species is rising. Relatively speaking, very much longer! Life expectancy in the Middle Ages, from approximately 300 to 1000 A.D., was estimated at about fifteen years; from 1000 to 1500 A.D. at about twenty years; from 1500 to 1700 at about thirty-five years; and as recently as 1900, life expectancy was about forty years. By 1993, however, life expectancy had risen to seventy-five years. By 2020, life expectancy should be more than double what it was in 1900—the greatest increase in recorded history. And this pace is expected to continue. As a result, increasing numbers of Americans are reaching the eighth, ninth, tenth, eleventh, and, yes, even twelfth decades of life.

Until now, world attention has been focused on the problem of explosive population growth. From a policymaking standpoint, a more critical phenomenon will soon steal the spotlight from population growth: population aging. Attitudes toward aging and the aged are being modified to address the demands of a much larger and far more diverse older population.

In my research on aging, I have also found good news about mental acuity. As it turns out, research says we lose mental capacity mostly because we expect to do so. As we age, we tend to demand less and less of our brains. We think we're too old to go to school, too mature to play word games, or too tired to embark on a new career. Like our bodies, our minds lose fitness with lack of use. Recent programs in France take direct aim at revitalizing aging people's brains. They are not only enormously popular but documentably successful. People can regain and even exceed previous mental capabilities.

Many of us are going to be around longer than we think. But are we sure we want to be? Most of our apprehension about aging stems from its traditional association with death. By today's definition, aging is anticipatory dying. This anticipation is promoted by biological, cultural, and social factors. American society is obsessed with youth and youthfulness; whole industries aggressively market products alleged to make you "stay young" (although nearly all, if not all, of these products are fraudulent). To be old in such a culture is to be categorized as an undesirable, as someone just standing in line to die.

But we can educate ourselves about what aging really is and what it isn't. Aging is a continuum begun at birth; it is not exclusive to those over forty. Old age is not a rehearsal for death. Aging is more than mere survival.

This book will help you revolutionize your vision of, and thereby your strategy for, your own aging and death. It is written today for today—to help people deal with seemingly overwhelming forces. The strategies it outlines for living long and dying fast are based on new facts about aging. Described in detail in the following chapters are a number of practices that can increase your probability of enjoying a long, healthy life. The topics covered include:

Exercise

No less than twenty laboratories in American universities are studying the physical and intellectual trainability of people over sixty-five. Improvement occurs at literally any age for both males and females.

Diet

We have more than enough evidence to prove that a

proper diet prolongs life expectancy in animals very closely related to ourselves.

Attitude

We follow the path of our expectations. We have allowed ourselves to gradually (sometimes rapidly) deteriorate in intellectual function. The psyche thrives on use; the mind and brain meet whatever demands are made on them. So make demands!

Sexuality

It lasts as long as you do. Don't allow it to disappear with age.

Human contacts

Maintaining relationships with other humans is an inestimable part of survival.

Smoking

Don't.

Sleep

Get enough of it. How much we each need is as variable as eye color.

Alcohol

Avoid it, except in moderate amounts.

Mental fitness

It's easy to maintain. Don't forget: You can remember. Education should be a life-long process.

Flexibility

Know your "sixth sense." Stretch daily to keep yourself flexible.

The aging game
Play it hard, and play to win.

Die? What, Me Die?

Nobody wants to talk about dying. We're just not sure about what happens after we die. Until it is necessary, we tend to avoid thoughts of our individual mortality. We need to come to terms with our mortality and accept that we all have a date with death—the only question is when. Once we accept the inevitability of death—and the pointlessness of delaying death by being kept clinically "alive"—we can begin to increase the likelihood of living long and dying fast.

My personal goal (and it can be yours, too) is to live as hard and long as I can, be as intellectually and physically healthy as long as I can, and die as fast as I can.

The rapidly expanding body of knowledge about aging permits me to do this, although I realize that most of the good news about aging isn't being shared. If, individually, we are finding aging to be much better than we thought it would be, we tend not to be aware that others are also discovering that it's really kind of fun. Do you wonder what it's like to be very old—between eighty-five and one hundred twenty years old? More than 70 percent of people in this age group report that they are in good health and happy spirits, do not feel lonely, and do not worry. Most lead lives of contentment and dignity. Family contacts are frequent, and personal relationships are a main source of joy. Only 3 percent either have no relatives or never see them. When centenarians wake to a new morning for the 36,000th-plus time, they do so optimistically, looking forward to a pleasant, active, and fulfilling day.

The Joys of Aging

Now that I have more rings on my tree than most, I enjoy the pleasures of being who and where I am. These pleasures come with a certain amount of accrued mileage. You stop doing things you don't like. You avoid someone you can't stand, rather than convincing yourself that it is your responsibility to be a nice person and muddle through. If you hate standing around at cocktail parties listening to people you hardly know talk about how much money they've made, you just stop it. Sometime in your maturation, usually later than you wish, you wake up with the glorious revelation that you don't have to do it again. You simply drop the invitation into the circular file and enjoy the sunset—ah, the silence!

You don't have to win all the arguments. A friend in his high seventies told me, "I still have vigorous, even passionate opinions, but I no longer have the need to argue with people too dumb to see it my way, the right way. When they bellow some totally wrongheaded notion, as though their entire ego structure depends on being right, I smile and say, 'Hmm.' Drives 'em crazy and saves my breath."

You become less concerned with appearance. You finally learn that comfort is preferable to style; in fact, comfort is style.

You have the joy of having been there, having bitten the bullets and fought the fights and learned the lessons. You've learned about love, the long-haul kind that gets deeper and richer as the years pile up. A marriage that outlasts the strains and changes. A friend or lover who knows all about you and still likes you.

It's fun to live long enough to see how everyone turns out. You see all your family and friends playing out the plot: The virtues, defects, and foibles of friends, relatives, and enemies lead to consequences, good and bad. You learn whether nice guys finish last, and how many cooks spoil the broth.

And, of course, you get to see your own drama unfold. Beginning today, make it your goal to keep the final curtain raised on that drama as long as possible, and then, when it's played out, to let the curtain drop quickly.

Part One

The Fountain of Youth:
You Are What You Ingest

Chapter One

Water:

The Universal Nutrient

Youth is the time of getting. Middle age, of improving. Old age, of spending: a negligent youth is usually attended by an ignorant middle age and both by an empty old age.—Anne Bradstreet

The only sure sign of life on another planet would be evidence of water. Water is an indispensable nutrient for all known forms of life. A fascinating fact is that all living things need the same concentration of water in their bodies to survive. The healthy adult human is 60 to 65 percent water by weight; so is the elephant, the mackerel, the bullfrog, the 'possum, and the dandelion. Only when you understand how this precious substance is used by the body, can you fully appreciate the concepts of health and disease.

To put it simply, your heart is at one end trying to pump all the water out of your body, while your kidneys are at the other end trying to hold it all in. If either succeeds, you die. Normal concentrations of minerals and other substances are maintained by drinking fluids and by excreting water and various chemical substances. A water-retaining hormone called vasopressin controls water excretion in your kidneys and sweating in your skin. Astoundingly, your kidney filters about 170 liters of water a day, but most of it is reabsorbed (about 169 liters, thank heavens). So we excrete only a liter or two of water as urine each day. In healthy young people, mineral substances and water are automatically balanced, thanks to an acute hormonal sensitivity to even slight changes in blood concentrations. At low blood concentrations, vasopressin is suppressed, allowing the excretion of a large amount of very dilute urine. When the mineral concentration is high, the amount of urine excreted is minimized by the "water" hormone.

As you age, this mechanism doesn't work as well; it becomes less responsive to changes in the blood. Several things are responsible: Thirst itself decreases; the kidneys become less responsive to vasopressin; and vasopressin secretion increases. Of these three factors, which can you do something about? Thirst! Even normally, thirst is experienced late in water depletion. By the time you feel thirsty, you are already dehydrated. This little-known fact is even more true as you age. Though you are fully capable of requesting and obtaining water, you will experience thirst less and less as you age.

One study explored the effect of twenty-four hours of water deprivation in active, healthy older men (sixty-seven to seventy-five years) compared to younger men (twenty to thirty-one years). The older men lost the same amount of weight but showed large increases in concentration of salts in the blood. Their urine analyses reflected inadequate excretion of salts. Nevertheless, the older men were not thirsty. In fact, all failed to correct their water deficit after two hours. Conclusion: People over forty, if left to their own thirst mechanisms, are likely to become dehydrated and to lose blood volume, even though they may appear healthy. People whose mental state has been compromised are particularly at risk. Many immobilized people with communication problems inhabit a virtual desert simply because they cannot ask for water.

Even for people without communication problems, dehydration is the most common age-related cause of health disturbances. It can lead to fatigue, a drop in blood pressure, perceptions of overall body weakness, and even fainting. Elderly people dehydrate easily in hot weather, but also during fever, infection, diarrhea, or vomiting. Many older people arrive in emergency rooms near death, not for lack of proper medication or care, but for lack of water.

Not only is water a necessary nutrient, it is also a catalyst for drug efficacy. All medications, liquids included, should be taken with a full glass of water. ("Water," by the way, does not mean coffee, tea, or juice. These beverages may contain caffeine or other chemicals, be high in sugar or calories, and interfere with drug action.) Drinking a full glass of water allows the medications to dissolve more quickly and be more readily absorbed, while reducing the possibility of stomach irritation. Thus, water—plain old water—can be one of the most useful agents for assuring proper drug action. In fact, most laxatives work because they are taken with plenty of water. Constipation follows insufficient water intake, and, therefore, laxatives simply do not work without enough water.

Many drugs, especially diuretics (which are used to treat heart failure), deplete body water volume. Unfortunately, many people report that they deliberately cut down on fluid intake to "help" their medications. They think that if their diuretic pills are supposed to get rid of excess water, then decreasing water intake will be that much better. But in doing so, they put themselves at risk of falling blood pressure, confusion, pseudodementia, and kidney problems.

Often older people ignore their thirst because drinking does not relieve persistent dry mouth or because they're afraid of becoming incontinent. Some nursing homes, concerned with inadequate water intake by their residents, ask doctors to prescribe four to six glasses of water a day for their patients. Once the order is written, nurses must give water, then witness and document the fluid intake.

Water, then, has many virtues:

- Water is the best diet drink around. If you are interested in losing weight, water gives the feeling of fullness with zero calories.
- Water helps reduce wrinkles. Well-hydrated skin is smoother and less prone to developing fine wrinkles. Water is probably the best anti-aging "vitamin" available for skin.
- Water helps the urinary tract resist bacterial invasion. By drinking water and keeping the kidneys flushed, patients prevent recurrent infections.
- Water is the only "medicine" that has no side effects!

What You Can Do

You must make an effort to drink plenty of water each day. To maintain optimum hydration, you should drink at least a quart of water (preferably two quarts) every day. Six to eight eight-ounce glasses of water a day are the minimum you should be drinking for good health.

Designer Water: Is It Any Better than Tap Water?

Once upon a time, when you went to a restaurant and requested water, you got a glass of ordinary tap water. Not any more. Ask for water, and the waiter recites a list of choices longer than the daily specials—water that comes from France, from Italy, from almost every spring and stream on the planet; water with minerals or without salt; water that sparkles or just sits quietly in your glass. When you ask for the wine list in New York's best restaurants, the waiters provide one for waters as well. Still, water is water, and designer water is no different than undesigned water. Actually, it may be of poorer quality than what flows from your tap.

The Muddied Image of Bottled Water

Not long ago, a batch of Perrier water was contaminated with the toxic chemical benzene, prompting a recall of 160 million bottles. This incident led to concern about bottled water in the United States. A year-long investigation of bottled water manufacturing practices ensued, with some surprising results. The General Accounting Office found that the Food and Drug Administration (FDA) had never adopted standards for contaminants in bottled water comparable to those for tap water, which are regulated by the Environmental Protection Agency. Yes, that's right. Bottled water can legally contain more toxic substances than tap water.

The General Accounting Office also found that the FDA did not monitor bottling facilities closely enough to make certain that bottlers complied with the few regulations that had been set. The FDA admits its regulation of bottled water is "imperfect," but they cite "no reason to question the safety of bottled water. The FDA considers bottled water to have a low potential for contamination or for causing sickness."

As it turns out, even the benzene-tainted Perrier water did not pose a significant health hazard. It is estimated that if a consumer drank sixteen ounces of the benzene-laced water a day, the risk of cancer would increase by only one in a million over a lifetime. In fact, there have been no complaints of any illnesses caused by drinking bottled water.

To its credit, the water bottling industry is beginning to regulate itself. Bottlers belong to a trade group called The International Bottled Water Association. Members voluntarily undergo yearly unannounced plant inspections by a nonprofit testing and certification organization known as the National Sanitation Foundation.

There is certainly room for improvement in the regulations regarding bottled water safety, but so far bottled water has caused no apparent health problems. Still, the General Accounting Office's report underscores the fact that, despite consumer perceptions, bottled water is no purer than tap water.

Bottled water consumption has quadrupled over the last decade in part because of its reputation for being purer than tap water. But about 25 percent of bottled water comes from the same municipal water sources from which tap water flows, though at three to twelve hundred times the cost. You may not mind this extra cost if you prefer the taste of bottled water, but don't think that you are safeguarding your health just because your water comes from a bottle instead of a faucet.

Chapter Two

Alcohol and Aging:
A Toast to Your Health

Millions of Americans will raise at least one cup of cheer at the end of the year, fostering that warm glow the holiday season engenders. Millions more will continue to drink the year round. While all these drinkers are risking their health to some degree, older drinkers are especially at risk. To understand why the dangers of alcohol increase as you age, you must first understand how alcohol works in your body.

Unlike any other food and drink, alcohol does not need to be digested or broken down by the small intestine. Alcohol molecules are small enough to pass immediately through the stomach into the blood. The alcohol concentrates in your organs in proportion to the amount of water they contain—the more water, the more alcohol. The brain has a high level of water because it has a high concentration of blood, which is about 90 percent water. This fact helps explain why alcohol affects the brain so strongly and why symptoms occur so quickly after drinking.

Alcohol leaves the brain slowly, much more slowly than it enters it. This creates a life-threatening problem in driving situations, not only because drinking impairs vision, judgment, and reaction time, but because alcohol also instills a false confidence. Drunk drivers believe they are more capable than they really are, and that their situation is safer than it really is.

Unhappily, nothing can speed up the rate at which alcohol is "burned off." It takes the body at least one hour to oxidize, or break down, a drink made with one-and-a-half ounces (a jigger) of liquor, a five-ounce glass of wine, or a 12-ounce can of beer. Contrary to popular opinion, cold showers, hot coffee, and brisk walks cannot make someone sober up faster. The best bet for anyone who plans to drink at a party is to leave the driving to someone who doesn't drink.

One reason alcohol makes you feel good is that it anesthetizes the centers in your brain that watch over your words and actions, putting to sleep the brain cells that control your inhibitions. These effects vary from person to person, and even within the same person at different times, because of such factors as

- how tired the drinker is
- the type of day the drinker has had
- the mood the drinker is in
- how much the drinker has had to eat
- what medications, if any, the drinker has taken
- the drinker's body size

If you think you can "hold your liquor," think again. Research shows that any driver's probability of causing a highway accident increases measurably at a blood alcohol level of 0.04 percent, which is well below the legal limit of 0.1 percent. A 180-pound man who drinks just two beers in an hour will have a blood alcohol level of 0.1 percent.

The physical effects of alcohol become even more pronounced over time. As you age, your total body water decreases, while your total body fat increases. Alcohol is insoluble in fat, so as body fat increases, alcohol tends to become more confined in the blood. As a result, older drinkers reach higher concentrations of alcohol in their blood sooner, and their organs are affected with greater intensity.

These increased concentrations of alcohol can damage nerve cell conduction. Some regions of the brain are more vulnerable to such damage, and, as a result, cognitive skills can be sharply impaired. Alcohol can damage mental alertness, diminish physical coordination, impair judgment, slow reaction time, and increase the risk of falls. In the long run, heavy drinking does permanent damage to the brain and the central nervous system. In fact, many symptoms attributed to aging, including irritability, inability to concentrate, and alteration in sleep patterns, are actually indications of problem drinking. Middle-aged and older people who drink, even moderately, are often diagnosed with dementia or some other organic brain syndrome, when, actually, they would return to normal if they consumed less alcohol. Incorrectly identified, such symptoms can lead to unnecessary and even dangerous treatment, including institutionalization.

The health problems associated with alcohol consumption are numerous. They include

- *cirrhosis*

  Cirrhosis is a hardening and contraction of the liver caused by long-term alcohol consumption. As few as three daily drinks for men and one-and-a-half for women can contribute to the development of the disease. Once it develops, it is irreversible, and the survival rate after five years is only about 50 percent.

- *coronary heart disease*

  Alcohol can damage heart tissue and exacerbate high blood pressure, a major risk factor for heart disease that afflicts nearly sixty million Americans. The greater the alcohol intake, the higher the blood pressure elevation. Alcohol can affect the body in unexpected ways, resulting in diagnostic difficulties by, for example, masking heart pain.

Some evidence does exist that moderate drinking—
one or two drinks a day—may protect against heart disease as well as stroke. But while heart specialists won't
complain if you are already having a drink or two a day,
they won't advise people to take up moderate drinking
as a preventive measure.

- *cancer*
  Alcohol consumption has been associated with a wide
  range of cancers, including those of the stomach, liver,
  lung, pancreas, colon, and tongue. Alcohol appears to
  augment the negative effects of smoking, increasing the
  risk for cancer of the mouth, larynx, and esophagus.
  Alcohol has also been linked with breast cancer. A
  Harvard University study of 90,000 women suggested
  that as little as one drink a day could increase a woman's
  chance of developing breast cancer by 50 percent.

- *problems of the immune system*
  Alcohol suppresses the immune system, making the
  body less effective at fighting infectious diseases.

- *infertility and impotence*
  The levels of male sex hormone are frequently low in
  alcoholic men. More than half become infertile and
  impotent after long-term alcohol abuse.

- *birth defects*
  Drinking during pregnancy is one of the top three causes of birth defects in the United States and the only
  absolutely preventable one. Mothers who drink alcohol
  during pregnancy risk giving birth to children who suffer from stunted growth, mental retardation, malformed
  facial features, or lifelong heart problems. Even women
  who have only a drink or two a day during the first six
  weeks of pregnancy (before they may realize they are
  pregnant) can produce children whose intellectual ability is impaired when they reach school age.

- *malnutrition*

  Because alcohol can depress the appetite and is comparatively high in calories, heavy drinkers often do not eat properly. (A gram of alcohol contains almost as many calories as a gram of fat, and over twice as many as a gram of carbohydrates or protein.) Absorption of food is also lessened by alcohol, which damages the absorption sites in the intestine, contributing to diarrhea, which itself exacerbates the absorption of nutrients.

Alcohol is a drug that interacts unfavorably with many other drugs (those sold by prescription as well as those sold over-the-counter). Drugs compete with alcohol for metabolic enzymes and chemical handling in the body, which causes the drugs to circulate longer in the bloodstream, thereby enhancing their effects. Drugs can also intensify the effects of alcohol, especially in older drinkers, causing more rapid and intense intoxication. When combined with the following drugs, alcohol can produce dangerous results:

- Minor tranquilizers such as Valium (diazepam), Librium (chlordiazepoxide), and Miltown (meprobamate)
- Major tranquilizers such as Thorazine (chlorpromazine) and Mellaril (thioridazine)
- Barbiturates such as Luminal (phenobarbital)
- Pain killers such as Darvon (propoxyphene), Demerol (meperadine), Tylenol (acetaminophen), and aspirin
- Antihistamines (both prescription and over-the-counter forms found in cold remedies and allergy medicines)
- Anticonvulsants such as Dilantin
- Anticoagulants such as Coumadin
- Anti-diabetes drugs such as Orinase
- Diuretics

Even moderate drinkers should check with their doctor or pharmacist about possible drug interactions with alcohol.

Alcohol abuse by older drinkers is much more common than is generally thought. Health professionals and the general public often ignore older problem drinkers because many of these drinkers have retired from public life and have few social contacts. Or, in some cases, families may even encourage drinking among their elderly members out of a misguided sense of deference and respect. But problem drinkers can be successfully treated at any age, as long as they are identified and diagnosed properly.

There are two basic types of problem drinkers: chronic abusers and situational abusers. Chronic abusers have consumed alcohol heavily throughout their lives. Many do not survive into old age; still, about two-thirds of older alcoholics do fit this category. Situational abusers have taken up alcohol later in life, usually in response to some traumatic situation: loss of income, declining health, the death of a friend or loved one. Situational abusers turn to alcohol for temporary relief but become addicted over time.

Of course, not everyone who drinks regularly or heavily is an alcoholic. So how can you tell who is? Not by the amount someone drinks. Because a person's tolerance for alcohol decreases with age, a person could be drinking less and still have a problem. Below are some of the symptoms that can indicate addiction to alcohol:

- Drinking to calm nerves, forget worries, or reduce depression.
- Losing interest in food.
- Gulping drinks and drinking too fast.
- Lying about drinking habits.
- Drinking alone with increasing frequency.
- Injuring yourself or someone else while drunk.
- Getting drunk more than three or four times in a year.
- Needing to drink increasing amounts of alcohol to get the desired effect.
- Frequently acting irritable, resentful, or unreasonable during non-drinking periods.

- Experiencing medical, social, or financial problems due to drinking.

On the bright side, problem drinkers and alcoholics who begin to drink later in life have an unusually good chance for recovery because they tend to stay with treatment programs. Help is available and can begin with a family doctor, a member of the clergy, an Alcoholics Anonymous chapter, an Alanon chapter (for relatives and friends of alcoholics), or your local health department or social services agency.

What if you suspect someone you love has an alcohol problem? How do you approach him or her? William Flynn, an Assistant Professor at Georgetown University's Department of Psychiatry suggests, "I tell the person, 'at one point alcohol was an extremely important part of your life. It did some wonderful things for you, but now you have to take action because it is no longer working for you.'"

If you must drink, limit yourself to one drink every hour and a half, or two to three drinks over the course of a four- to five-hour party. Sip rather than gulp, which gives the liver more time to process the alcohol. Experts say there is no simple way to determine when alcohol consumption becomes harmful. Their advice is not to exceed two drinks a day, a "drink" being five ounces of wine, twelve ounces of beer, or one to one-and-a-half ounces of whiskey, gin, or other distilled spirits.

Resources

- Alcoholics Anonymous is a worldwide voluntary fellowship whose goal is to help its members get—and stay—sober. The only requirement for membership is a desire to stop drinking. For information, call your local chapter or write to Alcoholics Anonymous, P.O. Box 459, Grand Central Station, New York, New York 10163. AA distributes free pamphlets on alcoholism, including one specifically written for older people, called "Time to Start Living."

- The National Clearing House for Alcohol Information is a federal information service that distributes written materials and conducts literature searches for the general public. For information, write the National Clearing House for Alcohol Information, P.O. Box 2345, Rockville, Maryland, 20852.
- The National Council on Alcoholism distributes literature and makes local referrals for treatment services. Call your local office or write to the national headquarters at 733 3rd Avenue, New York, New York 10017.
- The Food and Drug Administration distributes a wonderful article on alcohol and drug interactions, entitled "Liquor May Be Quicker, But...." A single free reprint of this article may be obtained by writing the Food and Drug Administration, HFE-88 5600 Fisher's Lane, Rockville, Maryland 20857.

Chapter Three

Nutrition:
Start Your Engines

Recipe for Youth
On the seventh day of the seventh month, pick seven ounces of lotus flowers;
On the eighth day of the eighth month, gather eight ounces of lotus root;
On the ninth day of the ninth month, collect nine ounces of lotus seeds.
Dry in the shade and eat the mixture and you will never grow old.
                    —*Yin Shan Cheng Yao, Chinese philosopher*

Do nutritional needs change with age? Yes. Human beings aren't like cars that can run on one type of fuel their entire lives. They must have different kinds of fuel at different periods in their lives. To appreciate how your body's nutritional needs change as you age, you must first appreciate how your body changes over time.

Scientists divide the human body into three parts: lean body mass (which includes bone, ligament, tendon, muscle, and cartilage), body fat, and water. On average, as people age, their percentage of lean body mass declines, especially if they do not exercise regularly. This loss tends to increase strikingly in later life. In many, it is compensated for by an increase in body fat, so that an older person's body weight often remains unchanged, or even increases.

Where is this lean body mass being lost? By age seventy, the kidneys and lungs lose about 10 percent of their weight; the liver, 18 percent of its weight; and skeletal muscle diminishes by 40 percent. Fortunately, a comprehensive exercise program can reduce or even prevent the loss of skeletal muscle.

Them Bones, Them Bones

Lean body mass is also lost through diminished bone density. Loss of bone density, or osteoporosis, begins in the early thirties. It affects many, if not all, parts of the skeleton. Until there is considerable loss of bone density, however, osteoporosis is symptomless. Osteoporosis accelerates after age forty, largely because of hormonal changes and lessened exercise. Women lose bone density more quickly if their ovaries have been surgically removed or if they have experienced severe hormonal changes during menopause. Loss of bone density is especially evident between forty and sixty years of age. Women lose an average of 25 percent of their bone density by age eighty, while men lose only 12 percent. Even trivial falls can result in vertebral collapse and fractures.

Many other factors can contribute to osteoporosis, some of which you can control, and some, you cannot. For instance, whites and Asians are more prone to osteoporosis. A person with a family history of osteoporosis is more at risk, as is a person with a small body frame (weighing less than 130 pounds). Physical inactivity is a strong contributor to osteoporosis. Smoking is known to accelerate bone loss. Having no pregnancies, strangely, is associated with osteoporosis. Young female athletes who train excessively and consequently cease to menstruate (amenorrhea) are more likely to develop osteoporosis. Early natural menopause accelerates bone loss; on the other hand, late onset of menstrual periods is also associated with bone loss. Milk intolerance, lifelong low intake of calcium, excessive alcohol ingestion, and consistently high animal protein intake (eating meat daily, as opposed to mixed types of protein in the diet) are all promoters of osteoporosis.

Many diseases are associated with bone loss as well: eating disorders such as anorexia nervosa and bulimia; hyperthyroidism; diabetes; liver and intestinal disease; rheumatoid arthritis; long-term feeding by stomach tube, various anemias, and a type of arthritis called ankylosing spondylitis. Many drugs can also contribute to the development of osteoporosis: cortisone, anticoagulants, anticonvulsants, diuretics, aluminum-containing antacids, tetracycline, chemotherapy drugs, and lithium. The most effective treatment for osteoporosis is prevention.

What You Can Do About Osteoporosis

Bone density is lost when calcium is withdrawn from the bones to fulfill other bodily demands. The following are things you can do to ensure that you have enough calcium and that it stays in your bones:

1. Adults should take in at least 1200 milligrams of calcium per day. This minimum is especially important for women over fifty and men over sixty. Taking four TUMS® (calcium carbonate) tablets a day will prevent a calcium deficit.

2. Protein intake also affects bone loss. Strangely, eating purified protein tends to increase urinary excretion of calcium, leading to osteoporosis. Eating moderate amounts of protein in the form of meat, however, causes no calcium loss, probably because of the dietary phosphorous in meat.

3. Vitamin D regulates the absorption of calcium from the intestine. Three mechanisms may be at work in altering vitamin D's role in calcium balancing and absorption:

- Vitamin D is hard to come by; its dietary sources are limited to a few foods.

- Vitamin D synthesis occurs in the skin and requires exposure to sunlight, but people tend to get less exposure to sunlight as they age. Skin may also become less able to convert sunlight to vitamin D over time.
- Conversion of vitamin D to its most active form occurs in the liver and the kidneys, organs that become less efficient with aging.

For these reasons, you need to be sure you are getting enough vitamin D and exposure to sunlight.

4. Regular exercise helps bones absorb and retain calcium.

Not All Calories Are the Same

Some systems—your immune system, for example—may become less effective with age, but there is encouraging research that suggests that the basal metabolism (the level of metabolic activity occurring at rest in humans) does not decline with age. In fact, the overall rate of protein synthesis and breakdown (a natural balance) has been found to be slightly greater in older men and women. The ability to process glucose and fats, however, does diminish throughout adult life. Thus, there is some evidence that metabolism becomes increasingly sluggish with age, although this change has not been systematically studied using our best and most current knowledge about nutrition.

What happens if you don't control your diet as you age? Let me remind you of the first law of thermodynamics: Energy can neither be created nor destroyed, but can only be transformed from one form to another. Nutritionally, this law is better stated as the energy equation: Energy in - Energy out = Energy stored. If you eat more calories (fuel) than you use, then the surplus energy will be stored as fat. So, to lose body weight, you must eat fewer calories (energy) than you expend, and your body will then burn the stored energy, or body fat.

Calories come from protein, carbohydrates, or fat. Carbohydrates and protein have four calories per gram, while fat has nine calories per gram—over twice as many! Weight loss (or weight gain) has more to do with the type of food we eat than with the quantity.

The higher the percentage of fat in the diet, the higher the percentage of fat in the body. If a diet is high in fat, it is high in calories. Calories that are not burned up as fuel are stored as fat. In addition, it takes much less energy to convert dietary fat into body fat than it does to convert calories from carbohydrates into body fat. As much as 23 percent of the calories of ingested carbohydrates goes to converting the nutrient to body fat, but with fat, only 3 percent is needed, so dietary fat is converted to body fat much faster.

Carbohydrates are like high-test gasoline. They are very combustible (digested and metabolized), and leave little waste. Carbohydrates are our most accessible form of energy for day-to-day activities. If we eat more carbohydrate calories than we burn, the excess is stored in a readily available form called glycogen. Glycogen is stored in muscles and the liver. This natural "gas tank" provides ready fuel of up to 600 calories—as many calories as in eighteen cups of spaghetti, twenty-one slices of bread, or thirty cups of bran flakes.

When your gas tank is full (that is say, when your glycogen stores are at their maximum), your body converts surplus calories from carbohydrates into body fat. This rarely happens when you are active and drawing on your reserves. The mechanism for storing carbohydrates as body fat is inefficient, and the high demand for carbohydrates as an energy source works in your favor. Generally speaking, only 1 percent of the carbohydrates you eat will be stored as body fat.

Unfortunately, there is no "gas tank" for dietary fat, so foods that are high in fat are simply and easily converted to body fat. Whatever is not burned as energy is stored as body fat. Sadly, even frighteningly, the amount of fat our bodies will store is limitless.

Early humans learned to store fat as a supply of energy for times of famine. These hunter-gatherers had to spread out over hundreds, even thousands, of miles to hunt game or migrate with the change of seasons. Their fat served as an efficient survival mechanism for them, but it is a mechanism we rarely need nowadays. We can find food year round without having to chase it down (and burn lots of calories in the process). We use many things other than our legs for transportation. The need for excess body fat as fuel no longer exists.

Look carefully at the next hundred or so Americans that you encounter. Americans are the champions at fat storage. (Too bad there's no money in it.) They produce body fat easily and in ample quantities. Coupled with an all-too-common sedentary lifestyle, Americans' love of high-fat foods has caused obesity to become a major health problem in the United States. Forty to forty-five percent of the calories in a typical American's diet come from fat, 45 to 55 percent come from carbohydrates, and about 14 percent come from protein. Presently, nutritionists are strongly recommending that 30 percent of calories or less come from fat, 55 to 60 percent from carbohydrates, and the rest from protein.

A happy consequence of a low-fat diet is that dieters can often eat as much as they want without exceeding their caloric maximums. "You can eat as much as you want and still lose weight?" Yes! Calorie for calorie, carbohydrate-rich foods take up more space in the stomach than do fat-laden foods, causing dieters to feel full on fewer calories. Some experts claim that the body eventually becomes less capable of storing fat. To reach this point, however, your diet must be well below 30 percent fat calories, and ideally less than 20 percent fat calories.

What does a high-carbohydrate, low-fat diet consist of? Foods such as pasta, rice, vegetables, and fruit; and protein sources such as lean meat, skim milk, eggs, and beans. This is very different from a typical American meal: a twelve-ounce steak with a small portion of vegetables and a large baked pota-to smothered in butter and sour cream. A high-carbohydrate, low-fat diet is made up of dishes such as spaghetti with clam sauce (hold the cream and butter) and stir-fried chicken with vegetables and rice. Carbohydrates (pasta, rice, vegetables, whole grains, fruits) should make up the main portion of your diet, not protein and fat. This kind of meal takes up a lot of space on the plate, making you feel that you're getting an ample serving. Avoid eating high-carbohydrate foods that are also high in fat: cookies, donuts, buttered popcorn.

Of course, you can approach this weighty issue from anoth-er direction. Exercising regularly and efficiently increases the output of energy and burns stored fat. Instead of reducing the input of energy (dieting), you increase the output (exercise) and lose weight by burning more calories than you consume. In this approach, weight is kept off more easily because the expendi-ture of extra calories (stored primarily as glycogen) prevents those calories from being stored as fat.

About 5 to 10 percent of the body composition of elite marathon runners is fat, yet they are able to consume 6,000 or more calories a day—three to four times what most of us eat. Runners must consume this large number of calories in order to balance their high daily caloric expenditure. With a high-car-bohydrate diet, excess calories never have a chance to be deposited as body fat. The vigorous daily workout depletes both glycogen stores and food consumed prior to the exercise. Any leftover calories are used to restore glycogen stores.

Combined with regular exercise, a high-carbohydrate, low-fat diet results in weight loss and an optimal body weight that can be maintained for years. The high energy cost of convert-ing carbohydrate to body fat, plus the constant withdrawal of glycogen supply from the gas tank for exercise, makes it diffi-cult to increase body fat.

One last formula for you: A gram is a unit of weight. One gram of fat contains 9 calories. If a food has 100 calories and 4 grams of fat, then the fat contributes 36 calories of those 100 calories, or 36 percent. If a woman eats 1600 calories a day and wants to be sure that less than 30 percent of the calories comes from fat, she can consume no more than 53 grams of fat a day. Confused? Thirty percent of 1600 calories is 480 calories. Since each gram of fat has 9 calories, it would take 53 grams of fat to equal 480 calories (480 calories divided by 9 calories per gram equals 53 grams). Try keeping track of how many fat grams you eat in one day. It's not easy to stay under 50, but that's what you should try to do.

For more information on counting calories and grams, consult the "bible": Nutritive Value of Foods (137L) is available for a small fee from the Consumer Information Center, Pueblo, CO 81009. This book lists 730 common foods, their caloric values, and their nutritional content (protein, fat, carbohydrates). Also listed are the Recommended Daily Allowances (RDA) for all major nutrients.

Of Fat Mice and Men

Obesity has been found to reduce life expectancy; thin people generally live longer. This conclusion is derived from weight and height tables based on insurance company statistics. Above certain "desirable" levels for different body builds, mortality rates rise with increasing body weight, particularly if the weight gain is mainly fat.

New data, however, raises the possibility that the greatest longevity is not associated with conventional desirable weights, but with levels 10 to 25 percent greater. Inordinately thin people have also been found to have reduced life expectancies. This observation may have nutritional implications for all adults; however, it does not take into account weight-reducing and life-limiting influences thin people may practice—for example, smoking and alcoholism—nor does it take into account the fact that people may become thin as a result of serious illness or injury.

If you lose extra pounds, then, will you live longer? Research on animals suggests that the answer is yes. In the 1930s, researchers at Cornell University found that decreasing a rat's caloric intake increased its life span. Similar dietary restrictions have lengthened life span in other species, too, including mice, fish, fruit flies, and rotifers (a microscopic animal). Other studies have concluded that life span (under experimental conditions) is inversely proportional to the amount of food eaten: The more you eat, the shorter your life. Keep in mind that most animals do not eat as they like in their natural habitats; perhaps all we can conclude from such studies is that free access to foods in the abnormal confines of a cage reduces survival, and that excess food intake and lack of exercise in humans probably does the same.

Most experiments that use dietary restriction to increase longevity begin with young animals. Experiments on the benefits of restriction of food intake after maturity are less common, but tend to show the same phenomenon—that it's never too late to repent.

Food restriction appears to increase life span by decreasing the rate of aging and delaying the onset of serious disease. Unlimited access to food may cause premature emergence of life-threatening diseases.

The progressive reduction of muscle mass and muscle strength normally caused by aging was slowed in test rats fed restricted diets as compared to control rats allowed to feed at will. Age-related decline in the responsiveness of fat cells was also retarded in animals on restricted diets. Blood cholesterol and free fatty acids were lower in animals on restricted diets. Old rats that ate at will showed increases in urinary volume, aging of tendons, ligaments, and joints, neuromuscular paralysis, and poor immunologic response. All these problems were absent in rats fed smaller amounts of food randomly.

But can we extrapolate these animal results to humans? Though these studies may appeal to a Protestant ethic of self-denial, there is little evidence that they hold true for humans: Undernourished, third world residents don't have the longest average life spans; the self-indulgent, overnourished people of the developed Western nations do. And studies of human beings suggest that being too underweight is as dangerous as being too overweight.

Nonetheless, animal studies do offer some evidence that nutritional intervention can favorably modify the aging process. Clearly, this is an area worthy of further exploration.

Nutrition and Aging

Most of what we know about the nutrient needs of older human beings is based on an extrapolation of the needs established for younger adults. In the United States, two age ranges have been established for determining the recommended daily allowances of nutrients for mature adults: from twenty-three to fifty years of age and over fifty. How ridiculous! It is unrealistic to presume that the nutritional requirements of a fifty-one-year-old are the same as those for a ninety-year-old. At best, recommended daily allowances are gross approximations. Energy needs change vastly from youth through old age. In addition, the increased incidence of chronic disease among older people complicates estimating their nutritional needs.

From a number of reports, it appears that we tend to eat less adequately as we age. A substantial percentage of the elderly population—perhaps as high as 50 percent—consumes less than two-thirds of the recommended dietary allowances for necessary nutrients, including calcium, iron, thiamine, riboflavin, niacin, vitamin A, and vitamin C.

Caloric intake also tends to decline with age. R. B. McGandy, a human nutrition researcher in Baltimore, reported a progressive decrease in average daily energy intake from 2700 calories for those between twenty and thirty-four years of age, to 2100 calories for those between seventy-five and ninety years of age. Only one-third of this decline was accounted for by reduced basal metabolism; two-thirds was attributed to reduced physical activity—a significant finding.

The same general picture has been seen in many other studies: A dietary research project in Scotland disclosed that younger male clerks (average age, twenty-eight) consumed approximately 3000 calories a day, while older male clerks (average age, fifty) consumed about 2400 calories a day, and a group of retired men consumed only 2050 calories a day. Similarly, young adult women in the study consumed an average of 2200 calories a day compared with just 1900 calories for more elderly participants.

A survey of inner-city residents in Syracuse, New York, over sixty-five years of age found that men consumed 1600 calories and women 1470 calories daily. A ten-state survey in 1972 showed that the average daily intake for poor blacks was as low as 1510 calories among elderly men and 1170 calories among elderly women. These figures were even lower than those reported in a survey of men and women in a Colorado nursing home: 1700 calories and 1300 calories, respectively. A 1971–1972 Health And Nutrition Examination Survey (HANES) of the United States population at large found that 16 percent of Caucasians and 18 percent of blacks older than sixty consumed fewer than 1000 calories per day. Among those whose incomes fell below the poverty level, these percentages rose to 27 percent and 36 percent, respectively.

Even allowing for the negative effects of poverty in these studies, it is apparent that energy intake declines with age. Absorption of specific nutrients also decreases. Identifying which nutrients are not being absorbed is critical because these decreases affect normal bodily function. One researcher noted that the overall energy intake declined from age 70 to age 80 by 19 percent; the most important factors in this decline were the frequent emergence of immobilizing diseases, voluntary immobilization, or general disabilities during this decade. We cannot conclude a cause-and-effect relationship between dietary deficiencies and diseases because we don't know whether nutrient needs really diminish with age or whether these other conditions preclude proper nutrition.

Specifically, what happens when food intake is reduced? Studies have found that many older people develop protein malnutrition: deficient intakes of iron, vitamin B1 (thiamin), folic acid, and vitamins C and D. In less privileged socioeconomic groups (such as those described in the survey above), the intake of thiamin, calcium, and iron has been found to be well below the requirements of recommended daily allowances. A study in Dalby, Sweden, showed that aging was associated with reduced consumption of folate, potassium, zinc, calcium, and magnesium. Persons living at home frequently had low blood levels of vitamin C (resulting in marginal scurvy), folate, and vitamin B12. Those in nursing homes had especially low blood levels of niacin and vitamin B6.

Do these deficiencies cause functional changes? Neurologic symptoms often are seen with such nutrient deficiencies in aging. Vitamin B1 (thiamine) deficiency, or beriberi, is associated with fever, and can precipitate an acute confusional state in some older patients (beriberi). Neurologic and psychiatric abnormalities can be precipitated by niacin deficiency (pellagra). Stress sometimes changes marginal nutritional status into acute deficiency, involving any of several nutrients.

A severe deficiency of vitamin C can cause scurvy, but even marginal vitamin C deficiency has been shown to contribute to early mortality. Vitamin C must be ingested because it is not manufactured in the human body. Vitamin C is absorbed less efficiently in older individuals, which strongly suggests a need for more vitamin C in older people, particularly nursing home patients.

Why does your total calorie intake decline with age? A. N. Exton-Smith has developed five possible explanations for the causes of malnutrition in general. The first is ignorance of the need for a balanced diet. This may be especially relevant to widowers who are unaccustomed to buying and preparing food. Among this group, for example, scurvy is more common than usual. A second cause is poverty, where a restricted range of foods is available. Third is social isolation, which tends to reduce interest in food and, therefore, levels of nutrition. For example, anemia and vitamin C deficiencies are more common in single men living alone than in men of the same age living with a relative. Fourth, a physical disability may contribute to malnutrition by, among other things, limiting access to grocery stores and restaurants. Older disabled individuals take in fewer nutrients than active people. Last, mental disorders, confusion, and depression become more frequent with age; these problems inhibit normal nutrition.

There may be other factors that reduce nutritional intake as people age:

- *disease*

  A number of diseases can inhibit the absorption of nutrients. The nutrients most often affected are the fat-soluble vitamins A, D, E, and K, as well as folic acid and vitamin B12.

- *alcoholism*

  Drinking alcohol contributes to malnutrition by substituting "empty" calories for more nutritional ones. Alcohol also interferes with nutrient absorption—notably, folic acid.

- *drug use*

  We tend to take more prescription and over-the-counter drugs as we age, and some of these drugs can interfere with nutrient absorption. For example, anticonvulsants can cause vitamin D deficiency, leading to osteomalacia or rickets.

- *increased protein needs*

  To maintain a healthy protein balance, we need more protein as our energy intake is reduced, especially when we are ill. Illness can cause losses of body protein stores. These stores need to be replaced from dietary sources. A high protein diet (intake that exceeds recommended daily allowances) may be needed during or immediately following an illness.

Appetite and Aging

Several factors can affect appetite as we age. One is the decline in our ability to taste and smell food. Loss of taste acuity occurs over a lifetime, and substantial defects in smell sensations are very frequent in the elderly. Recognition of food odors, such as cheese, orange, chocolate, and bacon, have been shown to be at least eleven times lower in people sixty-five years of age and older. Older people have fewer taste buds than younger people; whether this is due to poor nutrition and hydration is not yet clear. Oral cavity infections, poor hygiene, and diminished salivary flow contribute to difficulties tasting and smelling.

Loss of teeth can also diminish appetite. An estimated 50 percent of all persons become toothless by age sixty-five, and 66 percent by age seventy-five. The major cause of tooth loss is periodontal disease, which is sometimes an early manifestation of osteoporosis. Is osteoporosis a nutritional disorder? Certainly!

Many people grow up expecting to lose their teeth and their ability to chew, but advances in dental technology are such that all people can have fully functioning teeth in their old age. Some people, however, persist in using the same dentures they were given twenty years ago. Even dentures need updating. The shape of the mouth changes with time. Ill-fitting dentures can interfere with the ability to eat a normal diet, especially fresh fruits and vegetables and other highly fibrous foods that require a lot of biting and chewing. Poorly fitting dentures can irritate oral tissues, too, causing sores that make eating painful as well as difficult. Bad dentures detract from an otherwise attractive appearance, causing people to become uncomfortable eating with others.

A patient I know with Alzheimer's disease is a striking case in point. He lost all interest in food, to the point that he hid his meals to avoid eating them. His behavior was attributed to his compromised mental state, but when he was given a new set of dentures, his appetite returned. He began smiling at himself in the mirror and enjoying meals with others. Now his dentures will be checked annually, as anyone who wears them needs to do.

Could poor nutrition be causing some age-related chronic diseases? We don't really know. After ten years of residence in the United States, Japanese immigrants have less stomach cancer but more colon cancer than their counterparts in Japan. It has been speculated, but not confirmed, that increased dietary fat and decreased dietary fiber are to blame.

Whatever Did We Eat Before Oat Bran?

What about dietary fiber? For a generation, "fiber" has been a household word, carrying a remarkably persuasive aura of disease prevention. Cereal manufacturers in particular have touted the benefits of fiber. Now, many consumers rank breakfast cereals by the amount of fiber listed on the box, noting especially whether the cereal contains oat bran, a source of soluble fiber thought to be of special merit. But what is the truth about fiber?

Our ancestors consumed more fiber because their diet was made up of coarse foods, altered little by preparation. In more recent times, as wheat began to be milled into white flour, some decried the loss of fiber and bran. One New England clergyman who took up the cause was Sylvester Graham, who lent his name to graham crackers and graham flour, both with high fiber content. Graham was a fervent speaker who traveled widely, advocating making breads at home from coarse, unsifted flour.

Today's interest in dietary fiber is largely due to the efforts of two medical missionaries from the Makerere Medical

College in Kampala, Uganda. Drs. Burkett and Trowell were keen observers of the epidemiology of human disease. They described a scarcity of "Western" diseases in the Africans they treated. Their patients rarely had coronary artery disease, high blood pressure, diabetes, or such gastrointestinal disorders as constipation, diverticulitis, hemorrhoids, appendicitis, cancer of the large intestine, or hiatal hernia. From these observations, Burkett and Trowell hypothesized that the reason these diseases were rare in Africans was because their diet contained much more roughage that that of Westerners. They also determined, based on their observations, that the size and frequency of the bowel movements of a population are inversely proportional to the number of hospital visits. In other words, those who have larger and more frequent bowel movements are less likely to require hospitalization. While this correlation may seem amusing, it does suggest the health benefits of a high fiber diet.

High fiber diets are already being used to treat patients with constipation, diverticulitis, or hemorrhoids. Dietary fiber also helps prevent coronary artery disease by lowering cholesterol and blood fat concentrations, something oat bran supposedly does especially well. This is, in fact, why the bran war began. Is oat bran really better than other brans or fiber sources?

This question was answered by a study of oat bran published in the *New England Journal of Medicine*. Twenty normal subjects were fed one hundred grams of oat bran a day for six weeks, followed by six weeks of low-fiber wheat (white flour and cream of wheat). The results for the oat bran were as expected: cholesterol and blood fats were reduced. However, the low-fiber wheat diet also lowered cholesterol and blood fats. The researchers concluded that high-fiber grains and low-fiber grains reduce blood cholesterol equally well because both replace dietary fat with dietary fiber.

The bottom line is that there are far-reaching gastrointestinal benefits from a diet high in fiber, including the prevention of cancer of the large intestine, one of the most common cancers in the United States today. Researchers have been able to prevent colon cancers in laboratory animals by feeding them dietary fiber. They theorize that cancer-causing substances in the intestinal contents are diluted, bound, or rapidly passed out of the system by a diet high in fiber.

The Diet-Exercise Connection

In the 1950s and 1960s, the jogging craze was born. Dr. Kenneth Cooper and Dr. James Fixx were key figures in getting hundreds of thousands of people on the roads, jogging and exercising. At the same time, nutritionists, who were just as persuasive, were urging changes in our diet. Thus, two camps were born, championing two different life styles. "You are what you eat," said the diet advocates. "You can be born again through running," claimed advocates of athletic training. Exercise books gave lip service only to diet, and diet books made only passing mention of exercise.

Dr. Nathan Pritikin was a pioneer in reconciling these two points of view, emphasizing the connection between diet and exercise. This was not a new notion in medicine. Hippocrates had urged exercise and diet for his patients well before the birth of Christ. Sir William Osler, a famous American physician, teacher, and researcher, prescribed diet and steady exercise for his patients and students. In the 1950s, Paul Dudley White told James Michener, who was recovering from a heart attack, to avoid whole milk, eggs, and cheese. "Exercise to the limit of your endurance," he urged Michener, but also take a nap every day. Despite the efforts of such men, however, the general public remained largely uninformed about the benefits of diet and exercise. Many were unaware that high blood pressure and coronary artery disease could be controlled by diet and exercise. Through his residential programs, longevity centers, and books, Pritikin helped to bring the principles of diet and exercise to a larger audience.

Beware of Nutrition Quackery

"Lose weight while you sleep! No dieting. Eat all you want. The new super-grapefruit pill does the work for you."

Surely, you've seen claims like these before. They appear regularly in newspapers and magazines across the United States. Nutrition and health fraud are alive and well, thanks to the power of advertising. But isn't false advertising unlawful? Nutrition and health claims are regulated by the FDA. Unfortunately, the regulation just isn't sufficient. Only the most outrageous or life-threatening claims are investigated; the FDA has neither the money nor the staff to pursue every possible case. If a disclaimer (the fine print in which the seller denies any responsibility for the product) accompanies a product, the seller cannot be held responsible, even in cases of bodily harm. The FDA classifies nutritional supplements as foods, not drugs. For this reason, manufacturers do not have to prove the effectiveness of their product prior to marketing it. However, the U.S. Postal Service does require that mail-order advertising be truthful, and it is the primary mechanism for regulating and controlling mail-order nutrition products.

Nutrition quacks are successful because they appeal to our emotions, not to our logic. They lead us to believe in their "cures," relying on emotional testimonials of their myriad "cured" clients. Sensational tabloid newspapers and other media convey the quacks' false messages. Nutrition and medicine are not religions, they are sciences; the claims of nutritionists must be supported by scientific and clinical evidence, not by emotional testimony. The trouble is that quacks rush in where scientists fear to tread. When qualified health professionals cannot offer a scientific treatment for something, proponents of questionable therapies immediately step in because they are willing to say and do anything. They have no credentials and they are not monitored by any regulatory agency or licensing board. Dissatisfied clients have little, if any, recourse against such quackery except to avoid it in the first place.

Usually, unqualified practitioners diagnose the disease that they are pretending to treat as a symptom of some underlying disorder or toxicity. Cancer, for example, is often presented as the symptom of the problem rather that the problem itself. The real problem is the immune system. The body needs detoxification, and (or so it is claimed) that is just what the treatment will do. Responsibility for the cure is placed on the patient. If the therapy doesn't work, the customer feels that he or she, and not the treatment, has failed. This built-in guilt mechanism protects unqualified therapists from their disappointed clients.

Weight loss products and diets are by far the most popular items being promoted by fraud artists. Many of us crave an easy way to lose weight and keep it off. Promoters of diet books and diet aids all claim to know the secret to weight loss: foods, diets, pills, potions, and devices, all guaranteed to remove unwanted pounds and keep them off.

The FDA has banned many ingredients from diet pills because the makers of so-called weight loss products have failed to come up with evidence indicating that the ingredients really do help consumers shed pounds and keep them off. But this does not mean that weight control pills will be off the market. Exempt from the bannings are two of the most widely used diet pill ingredients:

- Phenylpropanolamine, an appetite suppressant commonly referred to as PPA, which is added to Dexatrim and similar products;
- Benzocaine, a local anesthetic used in chewing gum and fiber pills for the purpose of anesthetizing the tongue and the taste buds, thereby decreasing the pleasure of eating.

The FDA is reviewing the safety and effectiveness of these two substances. Even though the evidence suggests that they are unsafe, this is hard to prove. Experts say that the review process is taking much longer than necessary and that, at least in regard to over-the-counter diet pills containing PPA, the government should move quickly to limit consumer access. The potential for misuse of diet pills with PPA is high, especially for teenagers, a group who, most experts say, should not be using the drug in the first place. One survey of diet aid use among college students found that 40 percent of women and 6 percent of men had taken pills containing PPA. These users had ignored label recommendations about dosages and taken larger amounts than advised. Overdose of PPA can result in irregular heartbeat, constipation, insomnia, and dry mouth.

If PPA were a wonder drug, it would be easy to understand its popularity. But it is not all that effective. In one study, people on legitimate diet and exercise programs, supervised closely, lost only about a half pound more per week with PPA than without it. Other studies have shown that the drug does not promote weight loss among dieters who are already losing more than a pound a week. Despite the fact that a package of PPA-laced Dexatrim contains the words "lose weight fast" in large bold print, no research has ever shown that pounds will stay off once a dieter stops taking the drug. Thompson Medical Company, the manufacturer of Dexatrim, indirectly acknowledges this point in the literature that comes with the capsules. A brochure inside the box advises the user that "whenever you gain a pound or two, after you've reached your weight goal with Dexatrim, go back on the Dexatrim diet program. Don't wait until you've gained 5 or 10 pounds before you start to diet. Always keep a box of Dexatrim handy." This advice does more than suggest that people spend money; it also delays and distracts them from developing the healthy habits necessary to keep off weight—namely, a low-fat diet and regular exercise.

Proper diet and exercise will not only help you lose weight, but it will help you keep that weight off. Unfortunately, 95 percent of all dieters regain all the weight they lose. Real success at losing weight is a matter of permanent lifestyle changes.

To help you make these lifestyle changes, seek out a registered dietitian, a nutrition expert who can separate facts from fads, and translate the latest scientific breakthroughs into practical food choices. A registered dietitian has completed a minimum of four years of education and training in dietetics at an accredited college or university and has demonstrated competency on a national registration examination. You can find a dietician through your physician, local hospital, state or local dietetic association, or the American Dietetic Association.

Consumer groups and government agencies are also good sources of scientific information on nutrition and health. For example, the American Council on Science and Health is a consumer education organization concerned with issues related to food, nutrition, chemicals, pharmaceuticals, life style, environment, and health. The National Council Against Health Fraud investigates health claims, educates the public about deceptions, acts as a clearing house for people and organizations concerned with health disinformation, and supports legislation and legal action against health fraud. You can also call your local FDA office listed in the telephone directory under U.S. Health and Human Services. Every state has an Attorney General and a Consumer Protection Office that can be of service. If a diet program sounds too good to be true, it probably is. The bottom line on weight loss has never changed: When you use more calories than you consume, you lose weight. Regardless of what any huckster may claim, this single fact remains the indisputable, if unpopular, truth.

More Is Not Always Better

A large segment of our population is attracted by ads for vitamins and minerals implying that they improve your appearance, re-establish or augment your sex life, prevent or cure diseases, and lengthen your life. There is little scientific evidence to back up any of these claims.

Doctors do occasionally prescribe dietary supplements to correct deficiencies diagnosed in their patients. People who have osteoporosis (thin, brittle bones, subject to fracture) are advised by their doctors to take calcium supplements: calcium carbonate (such as TUMS®) often in combination with vitamin D and estrogen. Rigid dieters, heavy drinkers, and patients recovering from surgery may need some vitamin preparations and food supplements.

Too often people take high doses of many vitamins and minerals on their own, without a doctor's advice, in the hopes of preventing or curing a disease or lengthening their lives. This sort of self-medication is usually a waste of money. Worse, it can be harmful. Even something as beneficial as vitamin C can produce serious health problems when taken in excess.

We still have much to learn about the special nutritional requirements of aging. We do know that large amounts of vitamins and minerals do not seem to prevent or treat most health problems or slow the aging process. Too many people take multivitamin and mineral pills as a kind of "insurance" that their daily nutritional needs will be met. Multivitamin tablets taken daily are occasionally beneficial to people, but the value of any dietary supplement depends on many factors, including dietary habits and general health.

Excessive concentrations of some supplements can upset the natural balance of nutrients that the body normally maintains. Too much of certain nutrients can interfere with the effective action of other nutrients. Excessive amounts of some nutrients will fail to be absorbed and will pass out of the body, while other nutrients can build up to dangerous levels.

Megavitamins and high potency formulas are a real concern for scientists involved in nutrition. These supplements contain ten to one hundred times the recommended daily allowance for some vitamins and minerals. You may take them because you believe the RDA is only a minimum requirement, and that if a little is good, a lot will be much better. However, excessive doses of some nutrients can act like drugs, often with serious results. For instance, large amounts of vitamin A and vitamin D are particularly dangerous and can cause arthritis, headache, nausea, vomiting, diarrhea, and if continued over time, permanent liver and bone damage.

High doses of vitamin D result in kidney damage in adults. An excessive amount of supplemental iron can build up and be concentrated in the liver, damaging it as well as other body organs. Some supplements are of no value to anyone. One example is vitamin B15, or pangamic acid (calcium pangamate). This vitamin is sold in health stores as a treatment for heart disease, diabetes, glaucoma, allergies, and "aging." The substance is not needed in the human diet, and has no known medical usefulness.

Another useless and potentially harmful supplement currently sold in pill form is super oxide dismutase, or SOD. Scientists found that animals with long life spans have more of this enzyme in their bodies than shorter-lived species. This knowledge may someday lead to a better understanding of aging processes, but it is unlikely to lead to an "anti-aging" pill. SOD is a protein. When taken orally, it breaks down into component parts—amino acids—that cannot be reassembled. Therefore, SOD has no effect on body cells.

To dispel myths and win arguments with friends, write for two free articles, "Some Facts and Myths About Vitamins" (530L) and "A Primer on Dietary Minerals" (526L) from the Consumer Information Center, Pueblo, CO 81009.

Keeping in mind the evils of gluttony, use just enough food to keep Thee fit.—Sutra of the Sixth Patriarch

---

What You Can Do

Nutritional scientists have developed a list of nutrients essential to health, but no supplement contains them all; a well-balanced diet of a variety of foods provides all the necessary nutrients in the proper form. And there are other substances in foods that, though not essential for life, are beneficial to health.

You can get all the nutrients you require by eating a wide range of nutritious foods each day. A well-balanced daily diet includes at least two servings of milk or dairy products such as cheese, cottage cheese, or yogurt; two servings of protein-rich foods such as lean meat, poultry, fish, eggs, beans, nuts, or peanut butter; four servings of fruits and vegetables; four servings of breads and cereal products made of whole grain or enriched flours.

Occasionally, we may not get the vitamins and minerals we need from our daily diet. Digestive problems, chewing difficulties, dental problems, the use of certain drugs—all interfere with good nutrition. People with such problems may benefit from a dietary supplement.

If you are anticipating taking a supplement, ask your doctor or a registered dietitian if it's really necessary. They can check your health status and your diet and decide if steps should be taken to improve your nutrition. Do get such advice; a simple dietary change may be all that is needed. If you have been taking an unprescribed supplement, ask for advice about stopping it. It may be better to slowly reduce the supplement than to stop abruptly.

As you age, continue to educate yourself about medicine's latest findings about nutrition. Your body burns the fuel you consume differently as you age. If you weigh more than you want to, remember: The only way you can lose it is to have your calorie expenditure (work or exercise) exceed your calorie intake (eating). You can exercise more, eat less, or do both to lose weight. If you can't seem to keep or gain weight, aging may be nibbling away at your lean body mass, a potentially disabling occurrence. To halt this process, begin exercising and eating more and better foods. A high-carbohydrate, low-fat diet rich in high-fiber foods will stave off a multitude of ills, including heart and gastrointestinal disease. So start today: Eat lots of fresh fruits and vegetables, limit your fat grams, and exercise to keep your engine running cleanly and efficiently.

Part Two

Movement:
The Cure-All for Aging

Chapter Four

The Dangers of Going to Bed

Beneath the comfort of our bedsheets lurk a host of formidable dangers. When illness occurs, the usual prescription is bed rest. Hospitals are appraised by their number of beds. Doctors are assessed by their bedside manner. Severity of illness is measured by how long the patient is confined to bed.

Until the mid-nineteenth century, beds were used primarily for sleeping; only the very sick or dying were sent to bed. But since 1863, when a Doctor John Hilton in London wrote a book on the virtues of bed rest, it has been assumed that the first thing to do in any illness is to put a person to bed. According to Hilton: "If you put people to rest, God will cure them. Doctors are powerless without bed rest." Actually, immobilization is a curse. Doctors should think twice before ordering patients to bed.

Major deleterious effects begin within twenty-four hours after going to bed. Immobilization causes changes throughout the body, including multiple functional impairments and deconditioning. Bed rest also drastically increases the need for rehabilitation, often unrelated to the original disease.

What Does Bed Rest Do?

Bed rest affects every body system. Take the circulatory system, for example. In the upright position, gravitational forces cause blood to pool in the legs; normally, this pooling is countered by physical activity and motion. Within forty-eight to seventy-two hours of being confined to bed, however, the amount of blood pumped with each beat of the heart is reduced and the heart must beat more often to compensate. Rapid heartbeat and falling blood pressure are the consequences. People who have been in bed as little as three days have been known to faint on rising.

Fluid changes during bed rest can also cause fainting. Regardless of how much fluid a person takes in, increased urinary output occurs within twenty-four hours of immobilization. When this happens, the body's stabilizing mechanisms try to increase fluid volume by taking water from cells. Total body water decreases by about a quart and a half during a two-week bed rest. When attempts are made to get up and move around, reduced circulation from dehydration may contribute to fainting. An increased risk of blood clotting and anemia (low hemoglobin in your blood) are other consequences of dehydration caused by long-term bed rest.

The capacity for physical work diminishes as less oxygen is delivered to the tissues and oxygen uptake in muscles is decreased. Cardiovascular deconditioning from bed rest compromises oxygen delivery and reduces peak oxygen uptake, resulting in weakness and fatigue. In fact, 20 to 30 percent of muscle strength may be lost after only a few days of immobilization. Muscle mass decreases, oxygen transport to the muscles is impaired, and the range of motion of joints decreases simply from a lack of stretching. Because the integrity and strength of bones depends on regular weight-bearing exercise, bed rest can accelerate osteoporosis. Physical inactivity can also exacerbate compression of the vertebrae, injuring peripheral nerves and causing local paralysis.

Have you ever consoled yourself after an illness with the notion that at least you'd lost some weight? Unfortunately, little of such weight loss is due to loss of body fat. Most is due to loss of lean body weight and blood volume.

The body's hormonal and metabolic system are also affected. For example, the kidneys can easily filter excess calcium from the bones during periods of normal activity, but with extended bed rest, their filtering capacities can be exceeded, and the blood concentrations of calcium can rise to dangerous levels. The possibility of forming kidney stones from excess calcium in the urine is a real danger. After only three days of bed rest, the body's ability to handle sugar (glucose) is impaired; it takes two weeks, once bed rest is over, to normalize the metabolization of sugar. Bed rest decreases the body's production of the neurotransmitters that regulate normal central nervous system function. Male sex hormone has been found to be lower in immobilized men. And eight weeks of bed rest can alter levels of cortisone and thyroid hormone production.

Even basic functions like body temperature and breathing can be negatively affected by prolonged inactivity. Bed rest impairs the perception of cold and heat, lowers body skin temperature, and disturbs the balance between heat production and heat loss. Long-term horizontal positioning alters lung mechanics, air flow, and the volume of lungs; it can cause a 25 to 50 percent decrease in the ability to move air into and out of the lungs. Deconditioning of rib muscles and limitation of range of motion in the chest contribute to diminished lung effectiveness, resulting in a decreased ability to cough. In extreme cases, the lungs may collapse, or pneumonia may develop.

During long periods of inactivity, the immune and gastrointestinal systems also suffer. The white blood cells that should protect you from infection are compromised. Instead of improving your health, bed rest can actually raise your chance of contracting an infection, virus, or fungus. And prolonged bed rest can lead to constipation, compaction in the large intestine, and a generalized weakness of the entire intestinal tract. Use of a bed pan is as unnatural physiologically as it is socially, and embarrassment at performing private functions in an unfamiliar environment can foster postponement, which contributes to serious urinary and bowel problems.

Ulcers of the skin (bed sores) begin to form in as soon as six days. A combination of pressure, shearing, friction, and moisture creates sores that grow rapidly and heal slowly. Large ulcers may even result in infection, anemia from blood loss, and a drop in blood proteins.

Extended bed rest can induce psychological as well as physical changes. Because of a lack of sensory stimulus, brain waves actually slow down, and perception of sensation is reduced. During sleep, the length of periods of rapid eye movement increases (see Chapter 9). Negative emotions often surface, pushed up by the stress of inactivity. Most importantly, self-esteem is often reduced simply because an immobilized person is more dependent on others.

Even athletes are not immune from the negative consequences of immobilization. Professor Bengt Saltin, a famous exercise physiologist in Stockholm, studied the effects of immobilization in twelve highly trained, extremely fit young men: the members of the Swedish Olympic cross-country ski team. The men were all put to bed for twenty days, and their physical fitness was measured at the end of that period. Virtually, all levels of fitness had fallen by at least 25 percent. Professor Saltin reckoned that these very healthy young men had aged the equivalent of twenty-five years over twenty days—simply because they had been totally immobilized.

So much for the common hazards of bed rest; there are many others as well. Clearly, confinement to bed is an anatomically, physiologically, and psychologically unsound practice.

Look at a person who has lain long in bed, and you will see a pathetic picture indeed: blood clotting in their veins, calcium draining from their bones, feces stacking up in their colon, bed sores seeping—and the spirit evaporating from their soul.

• • •

Teach us to live that we may dread
Unnecessary time in Bed
Get people up and we may save
Our patients from an early grave.

—R.A.J. Asher

Shall I Never Go to Bed Again?

Temporary physical immobilization may be required at any age. An astronaut in space flight, an ill patient who cannot rise, an accident victim in a cast—all these people are immobile to some degree.

Proper bed rest can comfort and heal, but only if it is combined with as much activity and movement as possible, either in or out of bed. Excessive bed rest should be avoided. The elderly are especially susceptible to the consequences of immobilization. Too often, they are put to bed for no good reason, sometimes before any problem has actually been diagnosed. Many of the changes that come with aging are similar to those that occur with prolonged inactivity. The elderly person confined to bed is in double jeopardy, for the combination of immobilization and age can be deadly. Without exaggeration, unnecessary prescription of bed rest for the elderly is a factor in longer hospital stays, greater hospital costs, and higher rates of disease and mortality compared to the young.

What You Can Do

For those who must be in bed, portable toilets should be employed as an alternative to bedpans. Deep breathing, stretching, and general exercises are mandatory for maintaining health. Such physical activities can prevent complications and hasten recovery.

Most doctors have revised their attitudes toward bed rest. Patients are now being encouraged to sit and walk the first day after a major operation. Women get out of bed hours after giving birth. Heart attack victims are up and walking again within days.

Is it safe to exercise when you are ill? A study done on sixty men, all over the age of sixty-four and all suffering from at least one chronic disease, suggests that it is. The subjects were asked to exercise for ninety minutes by riding a stationary bike, stretching, lifting weights, or walking. Forty-nine of the sixty-nine people completed the four-month program; weekly attendance averaged 69 percent. The study found that, on average,

- participants increased their time on the treadmill from 8.5 to 11.2 minutes
- resting heart rate decreased from 68 to 55 beats a minute
- hip flexibility increased from 59 to 68 degrees
- abdominal muscle strength also increased strikingly, without any major complications.

These results demonstrate that it is advantageous for older people, even those with chronic disease, to stay physically active. By avoiding bed rest and exercising regularly, seniors can retard the age-related decline in their aerobic capacity, improve the quality of their sleep, halt the wasting of their muscles, prevent osteoporosis, and generally improve their cardiovascular fitness, strength, flexibility, and self-esteem.

Chapter Five

The Sixth Sense:
Flexibility and Stretching

Youth, large, lusty, loving
Youth full of grace, force, fascination
Do you know that Old Age may come after you with equal grace,
force, fascination?
—*Walt Whitman*

Most of us know that we have five senses: sight, hearing, taste, smell, and touch. But not everyone knows that we have a sixth sense—a marvelous faculty present in every tissue in our bodies. Unlike the other senses, this sixth sense works without our even being aware of it, taking care of us in remarkably efficient ways. The sense is called "proprioception," and it is the unconscious perception of movement and spatial orientation arising from stimuli within our bodies.

In the 1890s, the great neurophysiologist Sir Charles Sherrington scientifically demonstrated the presence of this automatic nervous system for the first time. In all tissues of the body, but notably in and around the joints, he found special receptors that are stimulated when stretched by a surrounding muscle. A nerve attached to the receptor sends a message concerning the muscle's movement to the spinal cord and from there to the brain, where the information is processed. The brain then automatically responds with a message to the muscle, telling it what it needs to do to maintain bodily balance, adjust posture, or move some part of the body.

Throughout your body, hundreds of millions of these receptors are activated by even the slightest movement in their immediate tissue environment. Requiring no conscious intention, they continuously relay messages to and from your brain. Thus, it is no accident that as you sit reading this book you know where your big toe is. Your brain is constantly receiving signals informing it of the location and status of the structures in your body.

Does this system require maintenance? Does it change with age? The answer to both questions is yes. Over time, the amount of information traveling between the receptors and the brain can decrease, resulting in loss of coordination and equilibrium. If you don't take care of your sixth sense as you age, eventually you may no longer be able to make those instantaneous automatic corrections that are necessary to maintain normal balance.

Succumbing to social pressure as we get older, we tend to do less and less physically. The fancy word for decreased activity is "hypokinesis." The hypokinetic person inevitably loses flexibility. With increased sitting time, tightness develops in the flexor muscles: the upper arms, the upper legs, and the entire spine. Hip and knee flexor muscles are commonly tighter in older people than in younger people. This tightness is not an intrinsic part of the aging process but a consequence of relative or partial immobilization. Diminishing flexibility occurs at any age in any muscle that is kept in a shortened state for a long period of time. When muscles are not flexed or stretched, the proprioceptive nervous system loses its accuracy and speed, and, as a result, the likelihood of falling increases. Loss of flexibility in the joints, in turn, makes injury more likely when falls do occur.

Loss of strength and flexibility from inactivity inevitably leads to poor posture, which can develop into neck and lower back problems. Changes in gait inevitably result. The body develops a mild rigidity in the upper arms and legs, causing a decrease in overall body motion, fewer automatic movements, and a decrease in amplitude and speed. Walking becomes more uncertain, and shorter steps are taken to ensure safety.

Keeping Things in Balance

Twenty-eight to forty-five percent of community-living elders and 45 to 61 percent of elders living in nursing homes suffer falls each year. These falls are life-threatening events, particularly for those seventy years old and older. Some falls result in serious injury, including fractures of the thigh and upper arm bones, wrists, pelvis, and vertebrae. The frequency of falls increases with age, which can exacerbate general feelings of insecurity, resulting in a self-perpetuating cycle of decreased mobility and increased dependence.

According to large-sample studies, however, more falls are attributable to individual problems than to aging in general. These individual problems include the loss of the ability to control balance, weakness of lower extremities, partial paralysis, Parkinson's disease, Alzheimer's disease, blackouts, vertigo, depression, dizziness, cardiac arhythmias, epilepsy, and falling blood pressure. Sometimes a fall represents the first clinical evidence of an acute illness such as gall bladder disease or a urinary tract infection. Drugs can cause falling, particularly diuretics, tranquilizers, and alcohol. Impaired mental status, poor judgment, confusion, or disorientation have also been implicated. And at least 15 percent of falls are the result of external factors:

tripping on an irregular surface, slipping on a patch of ice, catching a toe on a fold in the carpet.

The truth is, healthy, active older people do not fall more frequently or for any different reasons than do younger people. Control of balance depends on a complicated interaction of many factors: vision, proprioception, body position, proper joint alignment, and the vestibular apparatus in the middle ear. Impairment in any of these areas reduces the ability to balance properly and increases the risk of falling, regardless of age.

> Age only matters when one is aging. Now that I have arrived at a great age, I might just as well be twenty!
> —Pablo Picasso

What is the relationship, then, between aging and impairment of balance? While it is true that postural sway (those small oscillating movements your body makes to maintain balance when you are standing still) is more limited in the elderly, most healthy elderly people are able to stand with both feet together, without external support, for at least thirty seconds. Healthy twenty- to twenty-nine-year-olds can easily stand on one foot for thirty seconds. Seventy- to seventy-nine-year-olds can do so for only fourteen seconds on average. Try it yourself. See where you "stand." Maybe you're better than you think you are. One thing I can promise you: No matter what your age, if you stretch daily and regularly activate your proprioceptive receptors, you will be able to increase the time you can balance yourself.

Researchers have shown that levels of proprioception decrease with age. An illuminating experiment found that elderly individuals were able to walk faster and more securely on a carpeted surface than on a smooth vinyl surface. Though this finding may seem odd, it makes sense if you consider how much more a carpet stimulates the soles of the feet than does smooth vinyl. The better people can feel the location of their feet, the easier it is to walk. For this reason, both healthy and disabled seniors should be encouraged to walk barefoot on a tightly woven carpet. An alternative is wearing shoes with thin, flexible soles. Running shoes, for example, combine excellent support, reliable traction, and a flexible sole.

As you age, your peripheral vision plays an increasingly important role in stabilizing postural sway. Healthy twenty- to twenty-nine-year-olds can stand on one foot with their eyes closed for an average of twenty-eight seconds, almost as long as with their eyes open. Healthy seventy- to seventy-nine-year-olds, on the other hand, can balance on one foot with their eyes closed for only about four seconds—on average, less than a third as long as they can balance with their eyes open. This difference illustrates seniors' increasing dependence on visual input to stabilize posture. The scientific data we have on the senses, however, suggest that our ability to train our senses does not diminish with age. Sometimes problems with balance and peripheral vision can be solved simply by providing adequate lighting, especially in hallways and stairs. Of course, persons with macular degeneration, cataracts, or other serious visual problems will still be at risk for losing balance and falling.

Nerves in the inner ear also play a role in maintaining balance. These nerves, which make up the auditory vestibular system, monitor head position and detect and act appropriately when the head moves about. Using both visual information and proprioceptive information from the legs and feet, the vestibular system channels all the stimuli necessary for controlling balance. If vestibular input is poor, loss of balance can occur, and evidence shows that the vestibular system does lose acuity with age.

Many researchers believe that there is a loss in the number of brain cells in both the central nervous system (brain and spinal cord) and the peripheral nervous system (including proprioceptive nerves) during the aging process. Nerve cells cannot replicate themselves like many other cells in the body can. Because of this, the nervous system is more vulnerable to wear and tear, and to mutations that may ultimately lead to cell death. Associated with age-related nerve cell death in the central nervous system is a 10- to 12-percent reduction in brain weight. Interestingly, when nerve cells are lost, branchings of the remaining live cells increase, which scientists regard as an adaptive response to the death of other nerve cells. Can such branching be encouraged? It appears so. Animals exposed to a rich intellectual and physical environment have much more branching than animals in less stimulating environments. Therefore, to optimize the function of your nervous system, you should design and maintain a stimulating intellectual and physical environment for yourself as you age.

Why do nerve cells die during the process of aging? Some researchers have suggested that nerve cell death is genetically programmed. Others blame nerve cell death on a reduction in the delivery of oxygen to the cells, or on simple wear and tear of the nervous system. "Wear and tear" signs include the accumulation of an orange pigment (lipofuscins). The lipofuscins are insoluble granular pigments that are thought to consist of unmetabolized waste from partially broken down membranes or other cell structures. Such wastes fill up the cell, causing it to work less effectively. Interestingly, lipofuscins don't accumulate to the same degree in all nerve cells; they are most often found in cells that are less active, or less frequently fired. For example, lipofuscins will not accumulate on the vagus nerve, a very busy nerve that is part of the parasympathetic nervous system. The trigeminal nerve, which controls sensory and some motor activity in your face and jaw, shows the earliest signs of lipofuscin buildup. It would seem that if we can keep our nerves busy by exercising our brains and bodies, we can avoid or delay this buildup.

The brain produces a host of compounds called neurotransmitters that direct the function of the nerves in your brain and body. The presence of these neurotransmitters decreases with age in certain parts of the brain. But again, with stimulation, brain cells seem to be able to overcome this decrease.

Sensory and motor impairments are present to a significantly lesser extent in older people who have involved themselves in a lifetime of physical activity and intellectual function. Maximum knee extension speed is similar for active individuals, no matter their age, but it is significantly slower in sedentary older people. Forearm movements of older athletes are significantly faster and more stable than forearm movements of sedentary elders. Grip strength is more impaired in inactive than in active older people. Clearly, physical and intellectual activities need to be a part of every person's daily routine.

Flexibility and Stretching

Flexibility is measured by the range of motion in a joint or group of joints. Range of motion is specific for each joint. Mobility in the hip joint has nothing to do with mobility in the shoulder; and the range of motion in one hip may be different from range of motion in the other hip. There are two basic types of flexibility: static flexibility and dynamic flexibility. Static flexibility is the range of motion about a joint without regard to the speed of movement. An example of static flexibility would be doing the splits. Dynamic flexibility is the range of motion about a joint while performing a physical activity.

A flexibility training program is a planned and regular program of stretching exercises that permanently and progressively increase the maximum range of motion of a joint or set of joints over a period of time. Such a program also increases the sensitivity and effectiveness of the proprioceptive nervous system. The benefits of a flexibility training program are practically unlimited. One benefit is muscular relaxation. If a muscle stays partially contracted or tightened for an extended period of time, an abnormal state termed "contracture" develops.

Contracture not only shortens the muscle but decreases its suppleness, its strength, and its ability to absorb the stress of movement. Thus, one flexibility goal is to relax the muscles.

Another benefit of flexibility is improved body shape. We all want to be attractive, and the best way to improve body shape is through a combination of diet and exercise. For body symmetry and good posture, stretching needs to be an important component of any fitness plan.

As an added benefit, fit individuals suffer very little low back or neck pain. Stretching also relieves muscular soreness, enhances physical and athletic skills, prevents injury, and is just plain pleasurable.

The benefits of stretching can be summarized as follows:
- Stretching promotes circulation, bringing more oxygen and nutrients to the muscles.
- Stretching prevents injuries. A stretched muscle resists stress better than an unstretched muscle.
- Stretching increases range of motion.
- Stretching improves body shape.
- Stretching loosens the mind's control of the body so that the body moves more automatically and autonomically. Proprioception is enhanced.
- Stretching makes running, skiing, tennis, cycling, or performing any sport or physical activity more efficient.
- Stretching helps coordination by allowing free and easy movement.
- Stretching reduces muscle tension and muscular pain.
- Stretching makes you feel more relaxed.
- Stretching develops body awareness.
- Stretching feels good.

Children tend to be more flexible than adults, and females more flexible than males. Body build also affects flexibility. The good news, however, is that flexibility can be improved at any age with appropriate training. While the rate of improvement will not be the same for everyone, everyone can benefit from flexibility training. Usually, aging is associated with a gradual decrease in normal muscular function: muscular strength, endurance, agility, and flexibility. But this decrease can be slowed (and even stopped) by a regimen of regular exercise.

How to Stretch

When done correctly, stretching feels good. Stretching should not be a contest to see how far you can stretch. Nor should you necessarily try to increase the degree of stretching each day. The key to proper stretching is regularity and relaxation.

Doing a stretch routine "cold," without warming up the tissues, is like starting a car in the morning and getting on the freeway without letting the engine warm up. You've seen commercials about engine wear. The same thing happens in your body. When muscles, tendons, and ligaments haven't been active for a time, they are stiff and more resistant to stretching. Joints that haven't been stretched don't have as much lubricating fluid between the surfaces of bone and cartilage, and are much more prone to injury. Active warm-ups are fundamental to any exercise program.

Regardless of age, anyone can learn to stretch. You need not be in top physical condition or have great athletic skill. Stretching can be done any time, even in bed. Sleeping under an electric blanket or down comforter warms your whole body, an ideal prelude for in-bed stretching exercises. Stretching can be done at work, in your car, while waiting for the bus or walking down the road. It's interesting to observe animals stretching; cats and dogs instinctively know how to stretch. They do so spontaneously, and they don't overstretch.

Stretching is easy to learn, but there is a right way and a wrong way to do it. The right way is a relaxed, sustained stretch held for at least twenty seconds, with attention focused on the muscles being stretched. Stretching rapidly, bouncing up and down, or stretching to the point of pain will do more harm than good.

Start your stretching easy—no bouncing. Stretch to a point where you feel mild tension. Then concentrate on relaxing as you hold that point. The feeling of tension should subside as you hold the position, so that you can slightly increase the degree of stretch. If the tension does not subside, ease off slightly and find a degree of tension that is comfortable. The notion of "no pain, no gain" does not apply to stretching. Correctly done, stretching is not painful; in fact, it feels good.

After easy stretching, move slowly a fraction of an inch further until you again feel mild tension. Keep the stretch under control. As tension diminishes, continue to increase the stretch gradually.

Do not hold your breath during stretching. Breathing should be slow, rhythmic, and controlled. To do a forward-bending stretch, exhale as you bend forward, and breathe slowly as you hold the stretch. If a stretch position inhibits natural breathing, then you are not relaxed. Ease up on the stretch so that you can breathe naturally.

The proprioceptive receptors near the stretch tissues are "fired off" in about twenty seconds, so keep track of the time you hold each stretch, being certain that you hold the proper tension for at least twenty seconds.

Muscles are protected from damage during stretching by a mechanism controlled by the proprioceptive nervous system. When you stretch muscle fibers too far (by bouncing or over-stretching), a nerve reflex is triggered, sending a signal to the muscles to contract. You have a similar involuntary muscle reaction when you touch something hot. Without even having to think about it, your body pulls away from the heat to prevent injury. When you stretch too far, you tighten the very muscles you are trying to stretch.

Getting Started

Although not an exhaustive list of stretches, the following routine will activate nearly all the proprioceptive receptors. Ideally, this stretching routine should be performed at least twice a day.

1. Standing with your head and neck in slight extension (i.e., looking at where the ceiling meets the wall), lower your chin to your chest, then start rotating, first to the right. Stretch as far as you can to the right side, then roll your head back, looking at the ceiling or as far back as you can. Continue the rotation to the left, returning down to where you started with chin on your chest. Repeat ten times. Then do this same rotation, stretching as far as is comfortable, but starting to the left side. Repeat ten times.

2. Keeping your arm straight by your side, slowly rotate your right shoulder, making as complete and large a circle as possible in a vertical plane over twenty seconds. Repeat for twenty seconds and then do the opposite shoulder. Alternatively, both shoulders can be stretched at the same time.

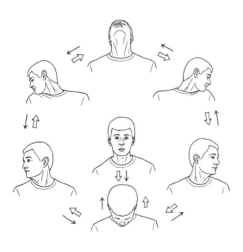

Stretch 1

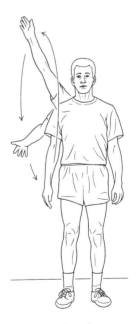

Stretch 2

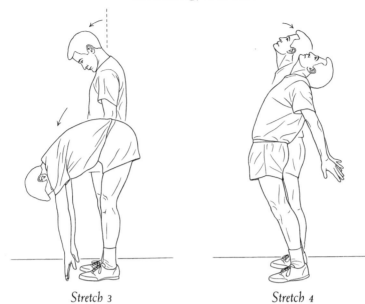

Stretch 3

Stretch 4

3. Keeping your chin on your chest, lock your knees and bend at the waist, reaching for the floor as far as you comfortably can. Hold for twenty seconds.

4. Lock your knees in the straight position, look up toward the ceiling, then arch your back as far back as possible, straining to extend your entire spine. Hold for twenty seconds.

5. Flex your neck to the side, bringing your ear as close to your shoulder as you can without lifting your shoulder. Then flex your whole spine to the side, reaching with your hand as far down the side of that leg as is comfortable. Hold twenty seconds. Repeat on the left side.

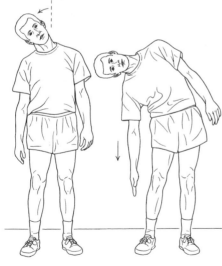

Stretch 5

6. While standing with your feet spaced one foot apart, rotate your head as far as possible to the right, keeping your shoulders square over your hips. After a few seconds, turn your shoulders and rotate your whole spine, looking as far as you can behind you to your right. Hold for twenty seconds. Repeat in the opposite direction.

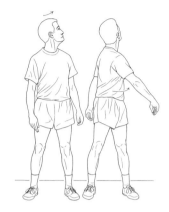

Stretch 6

7. Put your right hand up near your right shoulder. With your left hand and arm, push the right elbow upward, pointing it toward the ceiling. Keep your right arm relaxed in a passive stretch, letting the left hand cause the stretch. Hold for twenty seconds. Repeat for the left elbow, using the right arm to assist.

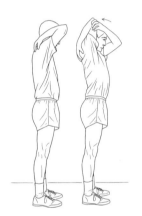

Stretch 7

8. Standing erect with your right arm straight at your side, reach behind your back with your left hand and grasp your right wrist. Lift your right forearm as parallel to the floor as possible behind your back. Hold for twenty seconds. Repeat on the opposite side.

9. Standing beside a table, kitchen counter, or chair, lift one leg and rest your heel on the surface—the higher, the better. Keeping your leg straight, lean

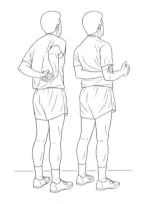

Stretch 8

71

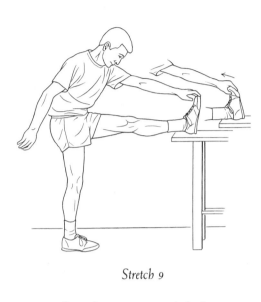

Stretch 9

forward, reaching for your toes on that foot. Hold for twenty seconds. Repeat on the opposite side.

10. Standing on one foot (using a wall or post if necessary to assist balance), grasp your right foot at the toes and bring your heel up to your buttock. Hold twenty seconds. Repeat with your left leg.

11. Standing on your left foot, grasp the toes of your right foot with your left hand. Using your right hand as necessary, lift your knee up and out as far as is comfortable. Your hip should be extended laterally. Stand as erect as possible for twenty seconds. Repeat the procedure on the opposite side.

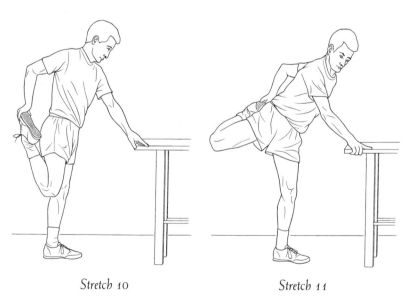

Stretch 10   *Stretch 11*

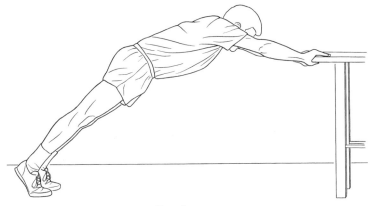

Stretch 12

12. Stand with your feet at least a foot apart and about three feet away from a counter or other stable surface. Put both hands down on the counter. Lean forward with your legs held straight, stretching the back of your calf as much as possible. Hold twenty seconds.

13. Spread your legs as far apart as possible, then reach for the floor. Hold for twenty seconds, stretching the inside of both thighs.

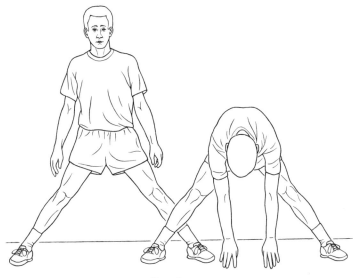

Stretch 13

73

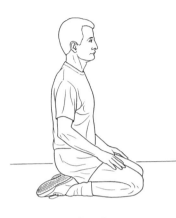

Stretch 14

14. Kneeling on the floor, sit back on your heels. Stretch the top of both feet and ankles. Move your torso slightly to feel the maximum stretch on the top of both feet. Hold for twenty seconds.

The evidence points in one direction: Use it or lose it. Level of activity is a critical variable in aging. The repeated use of the sensory and motor nerves helps prevent age-related loss of speed, strength, balance, and proprioception, and all but eliminates the threat of falling.

Chapter Six

Exercise:
A Catalyst for Longevity

Youth ended, I shall try my gain or loss thereby:
By the fire ashes, what survives is gold
And I shall weigh the same.
Give life its praise or blame;
Young, all lay in dispute;
I shall know, being old.

—*Robert Browning*

Exercise, smexercise! Don't you wish those self-righteous fitter-than-thous would get off your back? You'll exercise if and when you feel like it. What's so bad about not exercising, anyhow?

The truth is, it's risky—yes, even dangerous—not to exercise.

Without exercise, the condition of your body spirals rapidly downward. Bones lose mineral content and become brittle and weak. Muscles lose strength, and overall muscle mass diminishes. Consequently, it's easier to lose your balance, fall, and break your bones.

The Bad News

We tend to delude ourselves about retaining our youthful vigor, somehow sure that we will be the exception, the one person who remains fit with little or no effort. Sometime in our thirties, though, while performing a household chore or playing a game with the kids, we discover that no exception has been made. We simply can't do physical things as well as we could when we were younger. Whatever we may hope for as we age, we deteriorate if we don't exercise.

- About one inch of height is lost each decade after age fifty.
- Body weight, bone density, and muscle mass decline after age fifty-five.
- Shoulder and back muscles weaken, resulting in a humpback appearance called Dowager's Hump.
- Joint mobility and range of motion decreases.
- Rib cage elasticity diminishes, and the muscles of the chest and abdomen lose the strength to move air in and out of the lungs efficiently.
- Maximum achievable heart rate goes down, and cardiac output per beat decreases by about 1 percent per year. Each decade, general wasting occurs, and some 3 to 5 percent of actively functioning tissue is lost. The heart gradually must work more to achieve less. Ultimately, to perform even everyday tasks, all parts of the heart-lung transport system have to function very close to their maximum. The threshold at which the heart and lungs can no longer deliver sufficient oxygen to the cells is lowered.
- Flexor muscles shorten, and the muscles that support the head and the body in an upright position weaken. The shortening of muscles leads to skeletal changes that reduce blood flow, thereby decreasing oxygen supply.
- This decreased delivery of oxygen affects not only the muscles but the brain as well. Perception becomes less

accurate, motor responses grow faulty, and coordination, flexibility, and physical stability wane. So-called tonic neck reflexes and other mechanisms that help you walk, maintain balance, avoid vertigo, and judge movements, all begin to fade.

- The ability to lift and carry weights is reduced. Aging persons begin to lose independence and autonomy.

The Good News

Fortunately, this age-related deterioration can be slowed or even stopped with regular exercise. For example, one measure of fitness is VO2 max—the maximum rate at which a person can move oxygen from the lungs into the muscles, where the energy "fires off," creating movement. VO2 max declines about 1 percent a year after athletic maturity. With training, elderly subjects can maintain the same VO2 max over a decade or more, depending on how old they were at the start of the measurements. The ability to move oxygen does decline, but it can be maintained at surprisingly high levels into the seventies, eighties, and nineties. Any decrease in the level of exercise is matched by a corresponding decrease in the level of VO2 max.

Until recently, the science establishment presumed the physical aging process to be linear—a continual downward trend. But more and more evidence suggests that the aging process is not linear. A sedentary lifestyle may result in a continual downward trend, but even moderate amounts of exercise can change this slope to a series of plateaus. Seniors have it within their power and genes to stay in these plateaus. The harder they train, the better they are able to maintain desirable levels of fitness.

Okay, okay, so you really ought to exercise—but will you live longer if you do?

Based on what we currently know about longevity, human beings should be capable of living well over one hundred years.

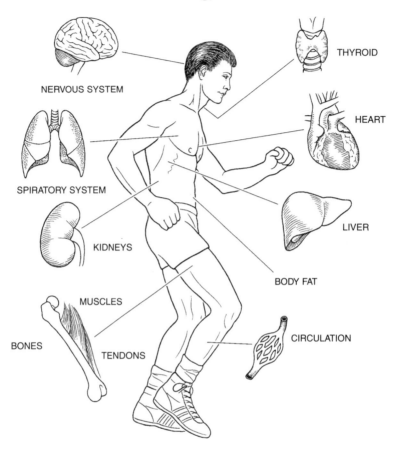

NERVOUS SYSTEM

THYROID

HEART

SPIRATORY SYSTEM

LIVER

KIDNEYS

BODY FAT

MUSCLES

BONES

TENDONS

CIRCULATION

Some Benefits of Exercise

Nearly every part of the body benefits from exercise: the nervous system, the lungs, the immunological system, the kidneys, the muscular and skeletal systems, the liver, the heart and cardiovascular system, and the hormonal system. All these critical areas of normal body physiology require exercise to function effectively and efficiently. And the functioning of all can be improved with exercise, not only enhancing overall health but extending longevity.

Past research on aging has tended to overemphasize age-related losses and neglect our vast heterogeneity. The effect of the aging process itself has been grossly exaggerated, while the modifying effects of diet, exercise, personal habits, and psychosocial factors have been sadly underestimated. We are not even close to living up to our genetic endowment.

For most of the last four million years, we were hunters and gatherers. We moved, literally, all our waking hours in the singular pursuit of food. We walked, ran, carried loads, built shelters, fashioned tools; we were as active as we could be. Then, quite recently in human history, farming and agriculture replaced hunting and gathering as the dominant mode of subsistence. Food (in the form of crops and domesticated animals) was now in close proximity, so there was no need to continue an intensely active nomadic existence. This was only the beginning of the decline of physical activity in human culture: Consider the difference in the level of physical activity between today's farmer and a paper-pushing executive.

This change in behavior has been so rapid that our genes have not kept up; we still have the programming to hunt and gather food all day. The closest that many of us come to living up to our genes' potential is an hour or so of walking in the mall on weekends. This, despite the fact that studies have shown that as little as half an hour of walking, gardening, or other moderate activity each day can significantly reduce the chances of dying from heart disease. According to one study, exercise, on average, added two years to the life spans of those over age eighty.

Swap Sweat for Serenity

Habitually sedentary seniors suffer not only from muscle deterioration but from a distorted image of their bodies. They perceive their bodies as broader and heavier than active seniors perceive theirs. Everyday activities seem more strenuous than they really are. Faulty feedback from sensory nerves misrepresents movement and body image. Consequently, these seniors feel clumsy and are fearful of physical activity in general.

As you age, you tend to lose the child-like pleasure in movement simply for the sake of movement. When is the last time you ran, rather than walked, out to your car in a parking lot, for example? Slowly but surely, you are reducing your movement. Eventually, older people become reluctant to move at all and may opt to remain in a chair or bed. The best remedy for restoring the joy of movement is movement itself. Exercise demonstrably reduces tension and provides profound emotional satisfaction. Exercise consumes free-floating energies and helps dampen aggressive tendencies or channel them into useful effort. And exercise improves the feedback between muscles and sharpens your sense of your own size and weight, thereby providing a more accurate body image.

Muscular movement is essential to the healthy functioning of the nervous system. As I pointed out in the previous chapter, there are anatomic structures in muscles, ligaments, tendons, bones, cartilage, and skin called receptors. The brain constantly receives messages from these receptors, alerting it to the position of various parts of the body. Signals are relayed through an area in the brain called the hypothalamus and back to the muscles to automatically coordinate movement. This sensory system is called the "sixth sense," or proprioceptive nervous system.

In addition to controlling the proprioceptive nervous system, the hypothalamus also influences emotional tone. Textbooks coyly say that the hypothalamus is involved in the "four F's": Fighting, Feeding, Fleeing, and Mating. Scientists now claim that positive emotions increase activity in the proprioceptive nervous system, while negative emotions decrease it. The converse may also be true: Muscular movement may stimulate positive emotions in the hypothalamus, thereby increasing proprioceptive nervous system activity. The happiest elderly people I know are all athletic to some degree, which seems to confirm this hypothesis.

Too often we think that it is normal for elderly people to feel depressed. But depression is not a normal part of aging. Indeed, it is the most common psychiatric problem among all age groups. Most older adults are not clinically depressed, but depressive characteristics are seen in the elderly more than any other age group. Fifteen to twenty percent of people over sixty-five suffer symptoms of depression.

The elderly may be more vulnerable to depression than younger people for several reasons. Age-related changes in brain chemicals and hormonal levels may be linked to depression. Also, the occurrence of certain diseases and the use of certain medications have been associated with depression, both of which tend to correlate with aging.

A considerable body of research now indicates that clinical depression is relieved in almost all individuals, including the elderly, after three to five weeks of regular exercise. A recent study of depressed people showed that their VO2 max, or maximum oxygen uptake, was unusually low. In another study, runners reported less anxiety and depression than people who were more sedentary. Still another study found that levels of depression declined in both depressed and normal subjects who jogged, played sports, or engaged in some other form of exercise. Those who ran most frequently (five times weekly) showed the greatest benefits. On the basis of these results, many doctors recommend that any treatment for depression should include vigorous exercise. Exercise is an effective and inexpensive alternative to antidepressant drugs, shock therapy, and sleep deprivation.

Some of the positive mental effects of exercise have been attributed to the exercise-induced production and release of hormones called endorphins, which are formed in the brain and spinal cord. Although endorphins are close relatives of opiate drugs, they are entirely synthesized within our own bodies, so there is no danger of addiction.

Before prescribing exercise, it is important to assess accurately both the type and severity of the mental illness. For instance, psychotic and schizophrenic people are not favorably affected by exercise. Nevertheless, there is little doubt that exercise generally contributes to good mental health.

A cautionary note: People who are on some antidepressant drugs should exercise with caution. Begin gradually with a fifteen- to twenty-minute, one-mile daily walk, increasing over a ten-day period to three miles in forty-five to sixty minutes. Most people are able to manage this schedule and maintain it.

Run Away from Diabetes

Over 14 million Americans suffer from diabetes. The most surprising thing about this statistic is that more than half of them don't know it. Nearly everyone with diabetes can improve their health by exercising.

Until recently, there was no direct evidence that exercise prevented diabetes. However, researchers from the University of California at Berkeley and Stanford University have lately demonstrated that physical activity can prevent the most common form of diabetes: non-insulin-dependent diabetes mellitus, or adult-onset diabetes. The researchers found that the incidence of this type of diabetes was twice as high among the least active subjects. They determined that for every 500 kilocalorie increase in energy expended per week, the risk of diabetes was reduced by 6 percent. (To put this into perspective: an average man weighing 167 pounds can expend 500 kilocalories in just one hour by jogging at a speed of five miles per hour, bicycling at ten miles per hour, or moderately swimming laps.)

Vigorous sports (swimming, tennis, and running) have a stronger protective effect against diabetes than less vigorous activities. All diabetics have increased risk of heart disease, disease of peripheral blood vessels, kidney failure, and blindness. Physical activity has long been prescribed for diabetics because it increases sensitivity to insulin. This increased sensitivity is especially pronounced in people at high risk—those with hypertension, for example, or those whose parents are diabetic.

The protective effect of exercise against diabetes is partly attributable to its benefits for weight control. Levels of physical activity and weight gain are correlated. And weight gain has been found to be a strong, independent precipitator of diabetes.

The concept that diabetes may be prevented by increasing overall activity, especially vigorous activities, is exciting. Anyone at risk for diabetes—persons who suffer from obesity or high blood pressure, or who have parents who are diabetic— should consider instituting a program of regular exercise. If the seven million or so undiagnosed diabetics would begin to exercise tomorrow, they might never need a drop of injected insulin.

Overcoming Aversion to Exercise

Do you ever feel like the only one who wants to exercise? When discussing exercise at work, do you feel that your enthusiasm is unique—that maybe you *are* the "exercise fanatic" your coworkers say you are? There are historical reasons why a large number of people are not only uninterested in exercise but even opposed to it. Many still believe that exercise can harm and shorten their lives. Where did this notion come from?

Aversion to exercise can be traced to a theory known as the Rate of Living Theory. This theory proposed that the faster you expend energy and use oxygen, the shorter your life span. Later, the General Adaptation Theory, developed by Hans Seyle, compounded the opposition to exercise in both medical and public opinion. This theory declared that vigorous exercise stressed the body, causing long-term, harmful effects. The consequences of exercise were compared to those of chronic infections, severe trauma, and disabling nervous tension.

Anyone paying even passing attention to science now finds these theories laughable. Not one study has shown that increasing energy expenditure has any deleterious effect on health. No research supports the idea that exercise causes the body to "wear out" or reduces life expectancy. On the contrary, it is now well established that, in contrast to machines, which wear out with more use, the more the tissues and organs of vertebrate animals are used, the more they gain in function. Exercise provides an essential stimulus for maintaining the structural and functional integrity of heart and lungs, muscles, bones, tendons, and ligaments, as well as the entire nervous system.

If You're Over 50 and Out of Shape, Can Your Body Still Become Fit?

Aging has little to do with a decreased ability to perform aerobic exercise; rather, as a recent study shows, the culprit is usually decreased physical activity. The study recruited two hundred twenty-four retired men, ages fifty-five to seventy-nine, with no significant differences in levels of fitness. The subjects were divided into two groups: One group walked and jogged three times a week, and the other group did no exercise at all.

At the end of a year, the men who were exercising regularly had improved in every fitness measurement taken. Their aerobic capacity, measured by VO2 max, had increased 12 percent over that of the group that had not exercised. Lung function, body weight, percent of body weight composed of fat, vital capacity—all improved at least 15 percent. The researchers concluded that even mild training could increase fitness in elderly men.

Exercise and Reaction Time

Reaction time is the length of time it takes for someone to react to a stimulus. A study of sixty-four male and female volunteers showed a gradual decline in reaction time with age for the sedentary adults in the group, but no corresponding trend for those who exercised regularly. Aerobic training appears to prevent the sorts of cognitive degeneration that would otherwise accompany aging—a finding that has practical implications for all sorts of activities, perhaps the most obvious one being driving an automobile. Exercise can help you retain the quick responses necessary for safety whenever you get behind the wheel of a car.

> **dawn**: The time when men of reason go to bed. Certain old men prefer to arise at about this time, taking a cold bath and a long walk with an empty stomach, and otherwise mortifying the flesh. They then point with pride to these practices as the cause of their sturdy health and ripe years; the truth being that they are hearty and old, not because of their habits, but in spite of them. The reason we find only robust persons doing this is that it has killed all of the others that have tried it.
>
> —Ambrose Bierce, *The Devil's Dictionary*

Does It Matter If I Don't Exercise Very Hard?

Two programs of physical activity for people over the age of sixty were designed to study variation in exercise intensity. Thirty-two volunteers over the age of sixty participated in a nine-week exercise program. The intensity of training for one group was maintained at 30 percent of estimated heart rate (low intensity), while for the second group, the intensity was maintained at 45 percent (high intensity). Both groups exercised for twenty-five minutes, three times weekly. Non-exercising volunteers were used as control subjects.

Though the group that exercised at high intensity had greater improvements in heart and lung measurements of fitness, those exercising at lower intensity also enjoyed positive changes in VO2 max. It would seem that even moderate exercise enhances fitness.

Yes, Do Sweat It!

Sweating is the body's principal means of cooling itself in hot weather. When sweat evaporates from the surface of the skin, the heat exchange results in cooling. Each liter of evaporated sweat removes 580 kilocalories of energy from the skin. What many people may not know is that this critical thermoregulatory function, on which most body functions depend, declines with age: you sweat less as you grow older.

In a recent study of the relationship between exercise, age, and sweating, forty male volunteers were separated into four subgroups of ten people each. One subgroup consisted of men who had exercised vigorously (at least one hour, four times a week) for the previous twenty-three years or longer. A second group consisted of older men who had been largely sedentary for at least the previous eighteen years. A third group was made up of younger men who had exercised regularly for at least three years and averaged over three and a half hours of vigorous running or bike riding per week. The fourth group was made up of young men whose habits were more sedentary.

Both of the groups who exercised regularly sweated at significantly greater rates than their sedentary counterparts. Researchers have concluded that lifelong aerobic exercise retards the decrease in sweating that typically occurs with aging. Only a few hours of exercise per week can significantly increase sweat release in older people. In other words, through regular exercise, you can improve your ability to sweat and thereby better regulate your body temperature.

Do Decades of Training Accrue Fitness Benefits?

When body composition, pulmonary ventilation, resting heart rate, blood pressure, and cholesterol levels of twenty-five champion American runners, between forty and seventy-five years of age, were measured, little deviation was found among the subjects under the age of sixty-five. At that point, however, these measures of fitness declined significantly. One hopeful finding of the study was that those who trained the most suffered the least decline in fitness. The question as to whether a lifetime of endurance training would show a less marked reduction in the measurement of fitness is still not answered. Surely, the great increase in numbers of the elderly in training will reveal more on this topic soon.

> Those who think they have not time for bodily exercise will sooner or later have to find time for illness.
> —Edward Stanley, Earl of Derby

Can Recreational Exercise Help Lengthen Your Life?

In Holland, eleven cities participate in a one-day, long-distance, recreational ice-skating tour. The popular event is held only if the ice is strong enough in the channels of Friesland, a northern province of the Netherlands. The first tour was held in 1909; fifteen tours in all have been held. The tour covers more than 200 kilometers. On the day of the event, parents leave their work and children, priests leave their parishes, doctors force colleagues to take their calls—life in the Netherlands comes to a virtual standstill.

The event starts in the dark at 5:30 a.m., and the participants depart in small groups every fifteen minutes thereafter. Control post officials watch the progression of all participants at each of the eleven cities, and controllers have the authority to order exhausted participants or those with signs of facial frostbite from the ice. They can also stop the race if the weather conditions become hazardous or the ice deteriorates.

Research was done to compare the long-term survival rates of the 2,259 skaters who have participated in the tour with those of the general population. The skaters had a much better survival rate. In fact, the faster their time to complete the skating tour, the longer they survived. The conclusions are obvious: People who are capable of prolonged vigorous exercise have a longer life expectancy than people generally. Recreational exercise is closely linked with longevity.

If You Were Once Athletic, Will You Have Any Advantage Starting Over?

The fitness levels of twenty-nine former athletes, between forty-five and seventy years of age, were measured at rest and during exercise. The subjects had all been successful competitors in endurance events before the age of thirty, but had been sedentary for at least ten of the years preceding the study. The study found that VO2 max of the former athletes was, on average, 20 percent higher than that of sedentary, middle-aged men. It was also, however, 25 percent lower than that of still-active athletes of the same age.

Why Some Older Athletes Can Outperform Younger Ones

Often, well-trained, elite older runners outperform younger, non-elite runners. One experiment sought to determine whether what was going on inside the bodies of young and old athletes was the same when they performed the same task. Master athletes between the ages of fifty and sixty were compared to runners aged twenty-two to twenty-eight. The study found that maximum oxygen uptake, or VO2 max, was 9 percent lower for older athletes than their young counterparts, despite similarities in performance. The master athletes also developed lactate release during steady exercise at a higher percentage of their VO2 max. (Lactate is a form of sugar that develops in the muscles during exercise when the cells receive insufficient oxygen.) Despite significantly lower VO2 max values, the older athletes performed as well as the younger runners because they were able to work closer to their VO2 max without producing any lactate for the entire duration of the race. Researchers have concluded that while there are differences between older and younger athletes, well-trained athletes compensate for aging so successfully, they can often outrace their younger counterparts.

In a similar study, sixteen highly trained endurance athletes, between the ages of fifty-nine and eighty-two, were compared to sixteen younger athletes. The two groups were paired on the basis of their training programs. Eighteen untrained, middle-aged men were then selected as a control group. Both groups of trained athletes had much better heart function than the untrained men in the control group. When adjusted for differences in body fat content, the VO2 max of the master athletes was found to average about 60 percent higher than that of the middle-aged untrained men. Maximum heart rate was 14 percent lower in the master athletes than in the young athletes. The major factor responsible for the lower VO2 max of the masters athletes was their slower heart rates. These older athlete's hearts worked less for greater energy output than their younger counterparts' hearts.

Exercise! How?

At least half of the losses in bodily function that occur between the ages of thirty and seventy are attributable to lack of exercise.

Regular exercise is the most effective way to avoid or postpone the mental and physical deterioration that comes with aging.

A Gallup poll reported that participation in fitness-building activities rose from 24 to 59 percent between 1961 and 1984. Unfortunately, 40 percent of the United States population do not exercise at all. Another 40 percent are active so seldom and to such a limited degree that they are not doing enough to avoid heart attacks. Only 20 percent of the population exercise enough to benefit their heart and circulation.

If you are out of shape, take heart. There is hope. If you have finally and irrevocably had enough of how you feel and look, if you are ready to rid yourself of your physical ills, if you are willing to follow the straight and narrow path of regular exercise, then make that leap of faith into a lifelong fitness program.

An effective exercise prescription is made up of four parts: (1) assessment, (2) motivation, (3) frequency, and (4) intensity and duration.

Assessment

Before you begin any exercise program, consult your doctor so that he or she can assess your age, general health, current level of physical activity, risk factors for heart disease, and personality before recommending a program for you. This assessment is especially important if you are over sixty, have a disease or disability, or take medication. Anyone who has been inactive for years should be especially careful, but everyone should enter a fitness program cautiously.

Motivation

Before choosing what kind of exercise you want to try, you must ask yourself, What types of exercise do I find interesting and fun? What attitudes, physical characteristics, and behaviors do I want to improve? Identifying these factors is critical for ensuring a life-long devotion to exercise. Ask yourself why you want to exercise...and get an answer. Reasons for exercising are not static; they change throughout a person's life. Don't hesitate to select a kind of exercise you like, or that you can enjoy at any skill level—walking or cycling, for example, as opposed to skiing or tennis. Strive for repetition, not gold-medal performance.

Those who have kept in good physical condition can participate in a much wider range of activities. Those who haven't should raise their general level of physical fitness before beginning a rigorous exercise program. The program you choose should be tailored to your ability, need, and interest.

Frequency

Fitness improvement requires at least three exercise sessions per week. Fitness experts say that if you work out three times a week, you can expect noticeable results in three to six weeks.

Intensity and Duration

The intensity and duration of exercise you can start with varies in proportion to your level of fitness at the start of the program. Exercising at 50 to 80 percent of your maximum heart rate results in improvement of all measures of fitness, but most notably an increase in the ability to move oxygen from lungs to the working muscle.

Beginning an Exercise Program

Once your current physical condition has been evaluated, then decisions can be made as to what activity will be best for you. There are four basic types of physical exercise: (1) aerobic or cardio-respiratory—the sort of exercise you get from distance running; (2) power training, in which maximum effort is sustained for only very short periods of time, such as running a 100-meter dash or swimming a 50-meter sprint; (3) anaerobic, or muscle-building, often achieved by lifting weights; and (4) flexibility or coordination training, including yoga and stretching. An ideal program would contain all four types of exercise.

Check your progress after the exercise program is underway, with the overall plan to continue it for the rest of your life. Any exercise program must have specific attainable goals and a record-keeping system to document progress. A sense of accomplishment is a prime motivating factor.

Start exercising slowly, especially if you have been inactive. Begin with short periods of ten to fifteen minutes, twice a week. Build up slowly, adding no more than ten to fifteen minutes each week. If all goes well, increase to twenty to thirty minutes, three or four times a week.

Be sure to include stretching, both before and after exercising. Stretching increases flexibility and creates a sense of well-being. Warmup and cool-down periods of fifteen to twenty minutes before and after exercise help tune up your body and prevent injuries.

Listen to your body: If you feel discomfort or pain, you are trying to do too much. Ease up, take a break, and start again at another time. Most people have no problem at all if they start exercising slowly. Consult a doctor if such symptoms as chest pain, breathlessness, joint discomfort, or muscle cramps should occur.

Finding an Exercise Program

Most American communities have centers where people can join exercise classes or other recreational programs. Inquire about fitness facilities and programs at your local church or synagogue, community college, civic center, park or recreation department, senior citizen center, service organization (Agency on Aging, for example), Jewish Community Centers, YWCA, or YMCA. Most of these centers offer organized activities for adults who have been inactive or who have health problems.

If you are employed—and I hope you are—ask about exercise programs where you work. Fitness improves performance on the job; many companies now provide opportunities for their employees to exercise regularly.

For free or low cost publications that describe exercise programs, write to the National Institutes on Aging, Exercise Building 31, Room 5C35, Bethesda, Maryland, 20205.

If exercise could be packed into a pill, it would be the single most widely prescribed and beneficial medicine in the nation.—Robert N. Butler, M.D., former Director, National Institutes on Aging

---

Skipping Rope and Rebound—
Good Aerobic Exercise

Walking and running are not for everyone, nor are they practical in some neighborhoods and in some weather conditions. Skipping rope is a good alternative. It doesn't cost much, and it can be done almost anywhere. Skipping rope develops heart, lung, and muscle endurance and improves agility, coordination, and muscular strength—all in a relatively short time. However, you need to be aware that the energy cost of skipping rope is high—too high for the average sedentary person just beginning an exercise program. You should be able to walk briskly for two to three miles or cycle vigorously the same distance before attempting to skip rope. Progress slowly with alternate bouts of twenty to thirty seconds of skipping, and equal or longer periods of rest. A person, already fit, might jump for about thirty seconds, do stretching exercises, and then do a longer bout of jumping rope. Good shock-absorbing shoes are important to avoid injury.

Another good alternative to walking and running is rebound exercise, which is done on a rebound trampoline. Exercising on a rebound trampoline is roughly equivalent to jogging a mile in thirteen to fifteen minutes. Like skipping rope, rebound exercise is inexpensive, can be done at home, and is effective.

Optimum Running

Efficiency is the key to optimum running. Running is a series of jumps, and the longer you stride, the faster you run. But there is more to running than stride length: You must also strive to get a high cost/benefit ratio for your effort:

1. Don't run with your hands. Rather, relax your upper body. Think of the lower body from the hips down as the horse, and the rest of you as the jockey. Your upper body provides breathing and balance. Only in a springing step do your arms become a factor.

2. Lean your upper body slightly forward so that the chest and head are just forward of perpendicular.

3. Breathe through pursed lips periodically to ensure belly breathing, which in turn ensures maximum movement of the diaphragm.

4. Lengthen your stride by pushing off, not by reaching ahead. The foot should not strike the ground in front of the knee.

5. Keep your buttocks slightly forward and push with them. Use your thigh and buttock muscles to increase the stride angle (the angle between the knees and pelvis).

6. Land on the ball of your foot, make heel contact with the ground for a millisecond, then push off. The more you can use your toes and the ball of your foot, the faster you can run.

7. Minimize up and down movement. Shoulders should move along a line parallel to the ground. This requires your knee to be bent when your foot hits the ground.

8. Eliminate crossover as much as possible. Each foot should land on its own side of a straight line in front of you.

> Your mobility is the next most important asset after your wits, so be aggressive in guarding it, promoting it, protecting it, and extending it.—Alex Comfort

Sociology of Exercise

As you embark on a new exercise program, you need to keep up to date on the current research on fitness. For instance, the pendulum of recommended exercise intensity is currently swinging toward moderation. This trend runs counter to the boom years of aerobic sports when the idea held that if a little exercise is good, then more must be better.

Research is also showing us that it may be more beneficial to participate in several sports or exercises than to be locked into one sport, which may lead to involvement at too great an intensity. Concentration on one sport increases the risk of an overuse injury; certain muscle groups are overused, others underused. For example, a switch to cross-country skiing in the winter is a wonderful complement to walking and running; it enhances upper body strength and overall flexibility. Left to their own devices, kids select different games all year round, and they do so because it's more fun.

Variability increases motivation for adults as well. We need to remember that exercise is a process, not an endpoint. Whatever we can do to make exercising more fun is desirable. Many adults find that social recreation is a good way to make exercising more enjoyable. "Social recreation" refers to activities which are done communally, such as playing tennis or racquetball, or running or skiing in a group.

Promoting Exercise at Work

As the work force becomes more sedentary and we learn more about the benefits of exercise, the need for workout facilities at work grows. Time, our most precious commodity, comes into play here, particularly as some authorities suggest that it is necessary to exercise at least three times a week. What is needed is something simple, cheap, and accessible. The provision of shower and changing facilities for office workers or laborers is the most cost-effective way to promote exercise and thereby better health. These facilities are especially welcomed by those who must drive to work or whose job does not entail vigorous exercise. This issue is important to the older population since so many of us are returning to work. We are often hired to positions of authority and control, and can promote these ideas.

Sir Roger Bannister, the Englishman who broke the four-minute mile, wrote the following words in the *British Medical Journal* in 1972:

> I can foresee a time when squash courts, recreation rooms, swimming pools, and running tracks will become a mandatory and integral part of any major new building; whether it be hotel, factory, condominium, or office block—as usual and necessary as modern plumbing.

In the last two decades, Bannister's vision has slowly begun to become a reality, particularly in the offices of larger American corporations, reflecting not only their approach to corporate life (which demands more and gives more to employees than in other countries) but also their enthusiasm for physical exercise. New York Pepsico's Fitness Director planned individual fitness programs for all 100,000 employees. The vigorous approach of the Xerox Corporation toward prevention of unfitness is now well-known.

Exercise for Reducing Stress at the Office

A brisk walk or a robust game of racquetball are popular prescriptions for reducing stress. But the office doesn't always come equipped with a racquetball court, and not everyone has the time or inclination to take a brisk walk. Fortunately, there are a number of exercises that can be done right at the desk. While few, if any, would advocate these exercises as a complete exercise program, they can help reduce stress and motivate sedentary people to start an exercise program. Deep breathing is a good beginning. Frequent stretching breaks are a healthy habit when your work requires concentration. You can concentrate on something only so long and be productive; productivity can be rejuvenated by stretching exercises.

Seated Stretching Exercises

Feelings of general well-being, alertness, and optimism follow systematic stretching. Workers who stretch two or three times in a working day improve their performance, both physically and intellectually. The firing of proprioceptive receptors, by the hundreds of millions, all over the body, is followed by an eagerness to get on with the work of the day. It takes about twelve to fifteen minutes to accomplish a fairly full stretch while seated at your desk.

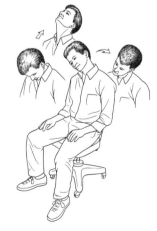

1. Sitting semi-erect, drop your chin on your chest, then slowly roll your head to the right, stretching backward to look at the ceiling, then rolling on toward the left. Stretching to maximum, return to your original starting position, chin on chest. Repeat ten times. Then repeat the whole stretch ten more times, but roll your head to the left first.

Stretch 1

97

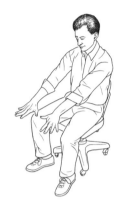

Stretch 2

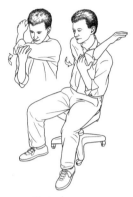

Stretch 3

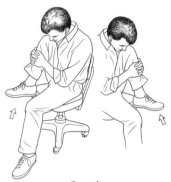

Stretch 4

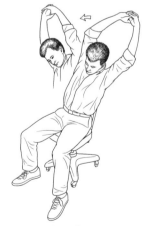

Stretch 5

2. Holding your hands before you, stretch and extend your fingers and hands as far as you can. Hold twenty seconds. Repeat five times.

3. Holding the left elbow with the right hand, push it sideways as shown, as far as you can, stretching to the maximum. Hold twenty seconds. Repeat on the opposite side.

4. Sitting, pull your right leg up toward your chest. Hold for twenty seconds. Repeat on the opposite side.

5. Clasping your hands with interlacing fingers, extend your arms above your head and stretch up to the right. Hold twenty seconds. Repeat to the opposite side.

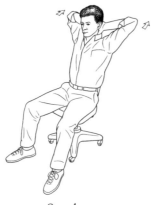

Stretch 6

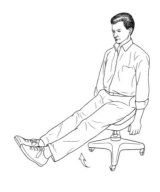

Stretch 7

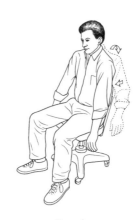

Stretch 8

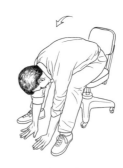

Stretch 9

6. Placing both your hands behind your head at neck level, with fingers interlaced, bring your elbows back as far as you can. At the same time, offer resistance by extending your neck. Lastly, gently rotate against the resistance, first to the right and then to the left, holding for twenty seconds each way.

7. Sitting, straighten both legs, making the thigh muscles as tight as you can. Hold for twenty seconds.

8. Sitting with your arms at your sides, shrug your shoulders upward and backward as far as you can. Hold the position for twenty seconds.

9. Sitting, lean forward as far as you can with your chin on your chest. Extend your hands and try to press your palms flat on the floor. Do it as far as you can. Hold for twenty seconds.

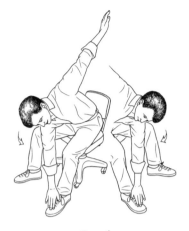

Stretch 10

10. Sitting, extend the left arm as far up and out as you can. Stretch it, then reach down with the right arm to the left foot. Hold twenty seconds. Repeat on the opposite side.

This series, if done well, will fire off the great majority of proprioceptive receptors, resulting in a general feeling of suppleness and optimism.

New Concepts of Fitness

Not many years ago the words "grandma" and "grandpa" conjured up images of rocking chairs, knitting, and pipe smoking. Today, some grandmas are playing competitive tennis, and some grandpas are running marathons. Until the recent boom in physical fitness, physicians had not steered older people towards sports or exercise; today physicians are being forced to change their attitudes about prescribing exercise. The concept of the older athlete has gained much credibility. There are many organizations of exercise- and sports-oriented people, both men and women, throughout our country.

For the past three decades the so-called "Leg and Lung" sports—running, in particular—have enjoyed enormous attention. But this focus is changing: Total body conditioning has begun to displace running in popularity. The foundation of any fitness program remains the aerobic component: cardiovascular and pulmonary fitness. But we have discovered that attention also must be given to strength and flexibility. I've seen too many instances of minimal fitness in the upper extremities, with great and excessive gains in the lower extremities, usually in compulsive runners. Even a soccer player, who needs strong legs and aerobic fitness, requires good upper body strength. Increased overall body strength makes sports performance easier and safer.

Exercise physiologists study the ways our bodies adapt to long-term training. Running by itself is inadequate training for masters runners who wish to maintain their aerobic capacity. Upper body lean muscle mass must also be maintained. Strength and flexibility training must accompany aerobic activity in a fitness program.

What is meant by strength training? Asking your muscles to work against some sort of resistance, usually a weight. Weight lifters are not necessarily the sweat-soaked musclemen you see grunting and straining on television as they lift hundreds of pounds of weights. Depending on your level of fitness, "weight" can be as little as one pound.

As we age, we lose muscle fibers. The less active we are, the more our muscles shrink and weaken. One study showed that 40 percent of women between the ages of forty-five and sixty-five could not lift ten pounds. Why does this matter? Who needs sinews in their seventies and eighties? Who wants to make that effort in their nineties? The answer is that being strong as opposed to being weak affects a lot of things: Without strength, everyday tasks such as hoisting a bag of groceries, pushing a vacuum cleaner, or lifting a grandchild will tire you. The less you are able to do, the less you try to do. This turns into a downward spiral as you limit your activities all the more.

The only way to increase lean body mass (muscle, tendon, ligaments, joints) is with exercise. Lift it or lose it. A program for achieving and maintaining muscle strength includes as many as fifteen different resistance exercises, using a number of different muscle groups, practiced three to four times a week.

So, pumping iron is not only for the young. Older people respond as well to muscle training as young people and enjoy the same benefits: more power, increased muscle bulk, greater freedom of movement. Strengthening techniques reverse aging's effects on muscles. For example, flexibility and strengthening exercises help prevent low-back pain. Most backaches are due to lack of flexibility of the muscles on the backs of the legs, combined with poor abdominal muscle strength and poor posture. Neck and backaches are rare events in older people who are fit. Weight training (plus a healthy diet and some aerobic exercise to trim fat) reduces the sagging upper arms and flabby bellies some people accept as a normal part of aging. As muscles gain tone, self-esteem shapes up at the same time. If you feel good, you act better and think better.

Strong backs, firm abdomens, lean arms, and sturdy legs help you function not only in normal situations but under abnormal conditions, too. Anyone of any age can compile great muscle reserve for times of stress, surgery, or injury. You are more likely to recover your health—and recover it more quickly—when you are in good shape.

Women and Exercise

Many women in their fifties and older were programmed during their formative years to become sedentary adults because inactivity was associated with femininity. Due to these influences early in life, older women in our society are much more likely to be sedentary than men.

In the current climate of greatly increased awareness of the benefits of exercise, even habitually sedentary older women can be motivated to initiate an exercise program.

Recently, studies of the relative physical capabilities of men and women have annihilated previous myths about male superiority. Slowly, all the myths about limitations on women's abilities are crumbling. A program of regular exercise can prevent or at least minimize many of the problems women are specifically subject to: heart disease, obesity, muscle weakness, and osteoporosis. Many symptoms of aging in women are more the result of a sedentary lifestyle than age, and can be reversed. A balanced program of aerobic, strength, and flexibility exercises helps to maintain and improve heart and lung fitness, control weight better than dieting, improve muscle strength, and reduce the risk of osteoporosis.

Every woman needs to take responsibility for her own health. A woman should consider getting a personal trainer for individualized instruction (if the expense of doing so is acceptable). Energy and strength will increase, not decrease. Life expectancy will be prolonged. Health care costs will be lessened. Aches and pains, tension and depression will be eased. The risk for osteoporosis, which is associated with "Dowager's hump" (rounding of the upper spine), loss of height, and tendency to fracture, will be significantly reduced.

One unfortunate consequence of aging, more common for women than men, is an increase in body fat. Excessive body fat is a problem not only medically but psychologically, aesthetically, and socially; but it is a problem that can be avoided. Many women believe that their fat accumulation began or increased with menopause, but there is no evidence that fat gain has any relationship to menopause. Another common belief is that with each pregnancy, the average woman adds weight that is not lost subsequently. Again, the increase in body mass experienced by the average woman over time has been shown to be the same whether she experiences pregnancies or not.

Fat distribution patterns are genetically determined, so to expect exercise to cause major changes in fat distribution is unrealistic. For instance, aerobic exercise promotes loss of abdominal fat more readily than fat at other sites. Abdominal fat is a risk factor for heart disease and diabetes, but fat on the outside of the legs is not associated with these diseases.

Women are often surprised to learn that the most common cause of obesity is inactivity. More fat will be lost by exercise than by dieting. The effectiveness of exercise in promoting fat loss results from several mechanisms: increased energy expenditure, increased metabolic rate, and altered body composition. One adverse effect of severe dieting (caloric restriction) is lowered metabolic rate. Resting metabolic rate correlates directly with percentage of fat; muscular women demonstrate a greater metabolic (fat-burning) rate than fat women of the same weight.

Women who suffer from a debilitating disease should also exercise, but they will require individualized programs. Women with arthritis, osteoporosis, diabetes, or other medical disorders should exercise in a way that promotes maintenance of muscular strength and heart and lung fitness. They can exercise muscle groups that are not affected by the disease, thereby strengthening the affected areas within the limits imposed by their disorders. Swimming is an excellent activity that women with most diseases can do.

Senior Athletic Movement

If you think that taking up a sport at your age is impossible, think again. You may not quite have the up-and-at-'em physical ability you once had, but you can still have as much enthusiasm. Remember that the genius of sports is not in brute strength but in the intangibles: intelligence and grace, technique and timing, heart and soul. The best football team is not the one that bench-presses the greatest weight. Good athletes are a dime a dozen, but athletes with character, intelligence, and experience are rare.

The media may not often cover such stories, but many athletes give their best performances later in life. Older athletes possess qualities such as skill and experience that compensate for the effects of aging. Age by itself should never limit athletic participation, for performance is often independent of age.

Anyone who aspires to compete in an athletic program should learn more about Masters programs. Competitors in these programs generally range in age from thirty to ninety, and are grouped according to age (e.g., thirty to thirty-four, sixty to sixty-four, seventy-five to seventy-nine). Wouldn't it be refreshing to enter a competition in which the only qualification was being old enough?

Below are the organizing bodies for these programs and competitions:

1. U.S. National Senior Sports Organization, 14323 South Outer Forty Rd., Suite N300, Chesterfield, MO, 63017. Phone: (314) 878-4900.

2. U.S. Tennis Association, League Tennis, 70 Alexander Rd., Princeton, NJ 08540-6399. (A national ranking program places players in competitions with others of their age and skill level.)

3. Athletics Congress of the U.S.A., Race Walking Committee, 36 Canterbury Ln., Mystic, CT 06355.

4. Masters Track and Field Committee, 5319 Donald St., Eugene, OR 97405.

5. Masters Long-Distance Running Committee, 5438 Southport Ln., Fairfax, VA 22032.

6. U.S. Masters Swimming, Inc., 2 Peter Ave., Rutland, MA 01543. Phone: (508) 886-6631.

7. National Masters News, P.O. Box 2372, Van Nuys, CA, 91404. Phone (818) 785-1895.

8. Masters Nordic Skiing, The Master Skier, P.O. Box 187, Escanaba, MI 49829.

9. The World Masters Cross-Country Ski Association, P.O. Box 5, Bend, OR 97709. Phone: (503) 382-3503.

Tennis (Absolutely) Anyone?

If you still doubt your ability to participate in a sport, I offer the following tips for playing tennis as a model for competitive sports in general. The creative finesse required in this sport can be applied to any sport with some thought and specific training for new skills.

- The best tennis players always let their racquet do most of their work, but this is especially applicable to older athletes whose stamina is limited. A wide-body racquet is more powerful and forgiving than a narrow-body racquet.
- Perfect your slice. This may have been a second serve in your past because you could hit it predictably and it wouldn't carry out. You're older and wiser now—start using your slice as an effective first serve. You will almost never double fault, and you'll drive your opponent crazy. Professional tennis players admit it's easier to return hard shots, and meeting a flat serve or drive is what most are accustomed to. They have to think how to return a slice.
- You may no longer be strong enough to hit the orthodox one-handed backhand with real power. So, learn the two-handed backhand.
- Of course you want to be as fit as possible, but sometimes your opponent is in better shape. So, return most shots as deep as you can down the center of the court. This reduces your chances of error and tends to make your opponent's returns come back down the middle. This strategy may allow your opponent to run less, but it does the same for you.
- Since you don't have a devastating service anymore, being the server is not an advantage. So, choose to receive if you win the spin of the racquet, and hope your enemy has a weak serve. If you're right, the first game will upset your opponent, giving you a headstart on winning the second game when you're serving. Concentrate more on breaking than winning service. Returning a serve that's not aggressive is the easiest shot in tennis—take the offensive.
- Play more doubles, where savvy counts for more than a

hard-hit ball. Find a compatible partner, and analyze your respective strengths. Who is the better server? The better net player? Decide which setup will work best for you when your team is serving. Start with that setup in your first service game, which will allow one extra game per set with your strengths where they work best.

- Be deceptive. For example, if your opponent faults on his or her first serve and are about to serve their second, move up quite far, making certain they see you do it. As they serve, pop back to your position. Fearing you're still there to smash their weak second serve, they will hit it hard and, hopefully, double fault. Or you might try varying your net position when your partner serves. This gives the enemy something to think about. If you move a step forward, they think you're trying to poach on their return and may angle that return too sharply to keep it away from you, hitting the ball out. Or they may try a passing drive down your exposed alley to keep you honest. Then they're in for a surprise because you never had any intention of poaching. Plan to move back immediately to cover such a passing shot.

- Opponents get used to your serve being the same every time, coming over the net the same way from the same place. So, vary your serving position. Most players stand close to the midpoint when serving from the right and out further toward the corner when serving from the left, making it easier to serve to an opponent's backhand. Practice putting the ball in from any position on the baseline. It will bother them to see you serving from a different place on the line each time.

If you fondly remember the satisfaction and fitness derived from a sport you played when you were younger, there's no reason you can't take it up again. Learn about new equipment and revamp your approach, incorporating the changes that have occurred in your body. Strategy is everything in sport, and you have years of experience—an enviable advantage no younger opponent can match.

Chapter Seven

Walking: The Best Exercise of All

It is day by day that we go forward; today we are as we were yesterday and tomorrow we shall be like ourselves today. So we go on without being aware of it, and this is one of the miracles of Providence that I so love.
—Mademoiselle de Sevigny

Some say walking in the 1990s is the jogging of the 1980s. It is, after all, the most basic form of exercise. Best of all, you need not learn how! The walking boom has produced many new terms: race walking, pace walking, power walking, fitness walking, health walking, rhythmic walking, mall walking, aerobic walking, even anaerobic walking for Olympic race walkers. You may ask: But I've been walking since I was one year old. What, all of a sudden, is "new" about walking?

The benefits of moderate walking are nearly the same as more intense activities like running and jogging. It takes longer, but the same changes occur. Walking is just less intense. You don't have to run a marathon to control your weight or get in shape. A typical man or woman burns about 120 calories either by running one mile or by walking a mile and a half. You can just walk a little farther each time, or walk more often to make up the difference, thereby achieving the same degree of health and fitness.

But what is really new is the realization of walking's many benefits and its universal appeal. Happily, walking is one of the few exercises to which age and physical condition pose no barriers. But don't underestimate walking. Very significant benefits accrue from brisk walking.

If you already exercise several times a week by running or weight lifting, you might think walking just isn't enough exercise to keep you in shape; these other forms of workout make you sweat so you know you're working. However, walking at a moderate pace brings a measurable response in fitness. James M. Rippe, M.D., head of the University of Massachusetts Exercise Physiology Laboratory in Worcester, tested 500 subjects. They reached their target heart rate by walking 4 to 4.5 miles per hour, three days a week. If you pursue a regular, scheduled program of walking, you can depend on seeing results in the long run, uh—long walk.

One great advantage to walking is that you can walk for a longer time than you can run. This feature makes walking a first-rate activity for developing muscle, bone, and joint endurance, as well as heart and lung efficiency. Because you can exercise longer, your metabolism stays higher longer, and your basal metabolic rate (the rate at which you burn fuel at rest) increases—you can actually lose weight while you sleep! The fitter you are, the more weight you can lose.

An even greater advantage derives from the pleasure most people take in walking. Sticking to an exercise regimen is the most difficult part of any fitness program. Walkers have a much lower dropout rate than runners, which enhances their long-term fitness potential.

In the United States, a million Americans sustain heart attacks each year. About half do not survive; many don't even make it to a hospital. Of those who survive, the majority may suffer no significant disability; cardiac rehabilitation programs are the reason for this. They make a big difference for these individuals, and walking is a primary part of all programs. All cardiac rehabilitation patients at the University of Vermont College of Medicine are placed on a progressive walking program as part of a total fitness plan.

Walking works miracles for many other serious ailments:

- All lung diseases are made less severe. Conditioning allows the lungs to accomplish more work with less shortness of breath. These changes are made permanent by following a walking program.
- Hardening of arteries in the legs is lessened by walking.
- People with the two most common forms of arthritis (rheumatoid arthritis and osteoarthritis) profit enormously by regular exercise programs; walking is far and away the best for these people. Joint stiffness and pain decline, while strength and power increase.
- Osteoporosis (bones that become thinner and more brittle, putting the person at risk of injury from falling), is favorably influenced by walking. It increases the density of bone. By walking regularly, you are at much less risk of falling and breaking a hip or wrist. Walking is the best way to slow down or arrest the bone loss process.
- Walking is also the most effective way of managing excess weight and keeping it off. This is especially true for obese people, who are at high risk for muscle and joint injuries if they begin running.

Walking is an effective option in a runner's training program. Many world-class runners include walking in their training programs. Walking on days off is useful. Injured runners are able to walk safely and can often avoid losing muscle tone when an injury necessitates stopping running.

Fast Walking

There is a big difference between strolling along at a couple of miles an hour and race walking at 8 miles an hour (about 7 minutes per mile). Walking for fitness requires a pace of about 3.5 to 4 miles an hour.

Many exercisers feel they must push until it hurts. For them, a painless hour of walking is too easy. The truth is, they are naive about walking's many benefits. Veteran athletes who take pride in their ability to push themselves to the limit are always surprised to discover the rigors of fast walking. Among them were ten superbly fit young men ages twenty-two through thirty-nine. In a study done in Dr. Rippe's laboratory, they reached and maintained their target heart rate for thirty minutes walking at five miles per hour. They found that this pace was more taxing than running. In fact, your body (if asked) would rather run. If you walk rather than jog at five miles per hour, it's a more difficult and meaningful workout and burns more calories: 125 to130 calories per mile for walking and 120 calories per mile for running.

This pace of five miles per hour is called "performance walking" (normal walking pace is about three miles per hour). Even highly trained athletes must work up to performance walking slowly. The muscle groups involved are the gluteus (buttocks) and anterior tibialis (shins); both are forced to work much harder than with other activities.

The next step up is race walking at seven and a half to eight miles per hour. To differentiate walking from running, the competition rules state that the walker's leading foot must touch the ground before the rear foot leaves it. The supporting leg must be straight when it is in an upright position. Arms swing and hips swivel for a thorough workout.

Race walking has long been an Olympic sport and, in fact, is the longest of all Olympic competitions: fifty kilometers or thirty-one miles. Some say race walking reminds them of the famous gait of Groucho Marx. Don't adopt Groucho walking unless you're going for the laugh instead of fitness.

Finally, those who are serious competitors in walking, do weight walking, which means walking with light hand-held weights. Whether weight walking is an effective fitness technique, though, is controversial.

Most people walk incorrectly, slumped over, with toes pointing outward, arms flailing, landing flat-footed. Biomechanically, the head and neck should be erect, shoulders relaxed, buttocks tucked slightly in, toes pointed straight ahead with feet spaced 3 to 4 inches apart, eyes looking five to six yards ahead. Walking with straight posture ("walking tall") gives the walker a higher center of gravity and a longer stride. Walking will convert Homo sedentarius into a vigorous Homo sapiens.

The figures below are rough measures of walking pace, based on an average woman's stride:

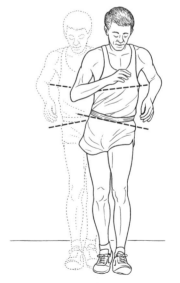

2.0 mph: strolling

3.0 mph: mild fitness walking

3.5 mph: errand-running pace

4.0 mph: average fitness walking

4.5 mph: fastest comfortable fitness walk, bordering on performance walking

5.0 mph: performance walking

7.5–8.0 mph: world-class race walking

The race walker here illustrates proper race-walking technique. Tipping with each stride is depicted by the dotted lines.

Are You Too Old to Start a Walking Fitness Program?

Most of your body's decline in function is not due to aging, it is due to neglect: failure to use muscle, bone, joint, tendon, ligament, and cartilage. The human body truly wastes away if not continually exercised—and this is true at any age.

At the Human Physiology Laboratory at Tufts University in Boston, gerontologist Maria Fiatarone, M.D. studied a group of quite frail nursing home women, all over age ninety. For a twelve-week period they participated in a well-instructed weight lifting program. All of them had a dramatic increase in strength, including a 200-percent increase in knee flexor strength. Can you believe it? No one is "too old" to be involved in exercise or strength programs.

> When grace is joined with wrinkles it is adorable. There is an unspeakable dawn in happy old age.
> —Victor Marie Hugo

Benefits by the Mile

Walking regularly conditions your heart, improves overall circulation, augments lung capacity, reduces blood pressure, and burns calories effectively. High blood pressure and obesity are very important risk factors for both stroke and heart attack. Walking affords protection against these killers.

Muscle strength is improved. Walking exercises most major muscle groups. This trims thighs and firms buttocks, by using the equivalent of over 2,000 leg exercise repetitions per mile. The rhythmic arm swing that naturally accompanies normal walking works chest, shoulder, and arm muscles. Proper walking in good posture strengthens abdominal and back muscles. This is achieved by keeping your chin up and eyes looking forward.

A journey of a thousand miles begins with a single step.
—Old Chinese proverb

One Foot after the Other

One of the great things about walking is that you don't need an instructor to show you how to do it—it is the most natural form of exercise there is. Something you do need is a good pair of walking shoes; most ordinary shoes just won't work. A comfortable, properly fitting pair of shoes is the most important equipment for a fitness walker. There are only a few genuine walking shoes available; both Nike® and Reebok® companies make walking shoes. But the company that has most seriously approached the designing of true walking shoes is the Rockport Company (72 Howe Street, Marlboro, Massachusetts 01752). I recommend their walking shoes.

Embarking on a serious program of fitness walking should be preceded by discussion with your physician. Your doctor may recommend consultation with a physical therapist to determine what kinds of muscle strengthening exercise you need. Someone with arthritis will profit greatly by physical therapeutic advice and education in walking.

Stretching exercises are highly recommended both before and after any walking exercise. Stretching loosens muscles for a longer stride and reduces the risk of soreness and injury. Some basic stretches are described in a brochure entitled: "Walking: The Exercise For All America." Single free copies are available with a business-sized, self-addressed, stamped envelope from: American Podiatric Medical Association, 20 Chevy Chase Circle NW, Washington, DC 20015.

There are three different walking styles, each with its own purpose and benefit. Strolling is slow and leisurely, the kind of walking you do as you admire the scenery or talk with a friend accompanying you. Functional walking is moderately paced, two to two and a half miles per hour, the kind of walking you ordinarily do as you go about your daily routine, with other goals and accomplishments in mind. Brisk walking is fast and steady, enough to get your pulse up to a fairly high rate. This walking is valuable as an aerobic exercise and one in which gain in strength and power is guaranteed.

A brisk walking program should be started slowly, perhaps 15 minutes every other day for a week. Then gradually increase frequency, length, and speed of the walks, always maintaining a reasonably comfortable pace. If you are breathing so fast that it is difficult to speak, you are working too hard. If joint pain occurs, try taking shorter and more frequent walks.

Gradually increase to at least thirty minutes, preferably forty-five to sixty minutes, at least four days a week. Many people, when they become involved in the program, find that it is interesting, instructive, and highly beneficial to walk every day. Incidentally, if you want to maximize aerobic benefits by figuring your target heart rate and the time you should be walking to reach it, a copy of the test is available: "Rockport Fitness Walking Test" from The Rockport Walking Institute, P.O. Box 480, Marlboro, Massachusetts, 01752.

Psychological Benefits

Without reservation, I can guarantee an improved attitude, greater mental alertness, and more positive self-image—even relief of psychological tension from a regular walking program. Walking allows an entirely different state of mind—almost a meditative experience. Walking can be a period of thinking new thoughts, practicing the art of thinking, letting your mind wander, reliving a happy moment, attempting to remember something you've forgotten—a philosophic period.

My observation is that both runners and walkers have high self-esteem. This may be induced by the release of neurotransmitters from the brain (hormone-like substances called endorphins), which induce a favorable psychological feeling. Self-esteem is a great possession. When little or no discrepancy exists between your actual self and your ideal self, self-esteem is there. The training of the mind, the art of thinking, and the creation of new thoughts are areas you can pursue, especially while walking alone. Use this time to contemplate the quotations of wise men and women:

- Jose Gasset Ortega wrote, "This I do know: No one else can do it for me. Man, every man, must at every moment be deciding for the next moment what he is going to do, what he is going to be. This decision only he can make; it is non-transferrable. No one can substitute for me in deciding for my life."

- George Sheehan, M.D., cardiologist, philosopher, author, and lecturer wrote in his 70th year, "I know I cannot stay young, but I can stay fresh. Though I cannot get younger, I can get better. Age brings problems—also solutions—with every disadvantage there is an advantage. For every measurable loss there is an immeasurable gain. Those are my thoughts for this new day."

Good stuff to think about while exercising.

Walking and Arthritis

Today's arthritis doctors appreciate the need for exercise—regardless of the type of arthritis or its extent. They realize that many of the symptoms and signs of arthritis in and around the joints are a consequence of failure to keep the joint moving to at least some degree. Ligaments and tendons lose tensile strength very gradually, capsules of joints become loose, cartilage tends to wear. All these are a consequence of what I call "stress deprivation" or "exercise deficiency": failure to achieve mechanical stimulation of all joint structures throughout the body. Of course, pain often restricts movement; but exercising up to whatever the limits are, under the guidance of a good doctor, can relieve and improve almost any patient with arthritis.

The optimism and attitude of the person determines whether he or she exercises to his or her maximum capability. I have seen many dedicated patients go from being extensively disabled to being quite functional. In many instances, the symptoms of the arthritis decrease in severity. Furthermore, mechanical stimulation of joints helps heal them.

Why Walk?

Walking is undeniably the safest way to achieve these medically proven benefits:

1. Walking is an excellent form of aerobic exercise.
2. Walking improves mood and mental function, as well as self-esteem.
3. Walking aids weight loss and keeps weight off.
4. Walking slows down osteoporosis (bone loss).
5. Walking relieves stress.
6. Walkers are less likely to smoke cigarettes than inactive people.
7. Walkers are more likely to follow optimal nutritional habits than inactive people.

"No pain, no gain!" Don't you believe it for a minute! It is a myth that you have to exercise very hard, i.e., that you have to hurt to achieve beneficial effects. Consistency in exercise rather than short-term intensity is important. Don't believe that walking is not intense enough to produce fitness. Of all the new scientific information about health benefits of aerobic exercise, most of the exercise studies have been done on walking.

In the 1950s, two studies linked walking to decreased risk of heart attack. London bus drivers (who got very little exercise) were compared to bus conductors (who walked up and down the bus aisles collecting fares, as well as climbing stairs on the London double-deckers). In a second study, postal clerks (who did sedentary work) were compared to mail carriers (who walked daily to deliver mail). In both studies, the walkers had many fewer heart attacks. Critics say, "How do we know the walkers weren't healthier when they started?" We don't. But even as circumstantial evidence, it cannot be ignored. Many other studies over the past two decades show that exertion during work decreases the risk of heart attack.

In the past three decades, a great deal has been learned about fitness in the human body: Exercise alone, though important, is not the only answer. It is just the cornerstone of a health care program. Maximum health implies improving flexibility and strength, improving nutrition, and lowering stress levels. Fitness walking is part of a total fitness program. Is walking as good as running, cycling, swimming, rowing, and many others? Yes! Walking is the safest, most practical, and most sensible centerpiece for a fitness program. It clears the mind and reduces stress. A daily fitness walk provides a break from work or boredom, and affords a period to sort yourself out or plan for the work ahead. These benefits are observable within only a few weeks.

The Exercise Tolerance Test

The exercise tolerance test determines whether or not it is safe to start an exercise program. In this test, you walk and then gently jog on a motorized treadmill at ever-increasing speeds and increasing grades. During the test, a physician examines the electrocardiogram (EKG) as your heart rate gets faster and faster. EKG changes help determine whether or not there is narrowing of the blood vessels supplying the heart (coronary heart disease).

The question often arises as to whether you need an exercise tolerance test. Any male over the age of forty who has been inactive for more than a year should take the test. The same is true for any female who has been inactive and is over age forty-five.

Running vs. Walking

The running (jogging) boom has resulted in significant and important benefits to American society, but it has also brought some problems. Running reminded us all of the importance of physical fitness; it drew us in large numbers into a healthy activity, decreasing our sedentary life style. People lost weight, quit smoking, and went on diets—all to the good.

However, running does place stress on joints and bones. Injuries frequently result, though rarely serious personal injury. The most troublesome difficulty with running is that it excludes so many people who desperately need to exercise. Many equip themselves with expensive clothes and running shoes and start a jogging program, only to become injured and discouraged in a few weeks.

Dr. Kenneth Cooper, president and owner of the Dallas, Texas Aerobic Center, spearheaded the practice of aerobic training. Nevertheless, he recently said that anyone who runs more than fifteen to twenty miles a week is surely doing it for reasons other than fitness. The *New England Journal of Medicine* published an article describing "Obligate Runners," people who run up to one hundred miles a week in spite of injury or joint abnormalities (these are a small minority to be sure). National surveys have shown the average fitness level of Americans has declined over the past ten years despite the running boom. This is where fitness walking comes in. Very simply, fitness walking is the best exercise for the great majority of Americans.

Lifetime Exercise

Short-term conditioning programs are just what they say: short term. Health benefits of exercise accumulate over a lifetime and fitness walking is the perfect sport for such training. Many Americans are increasingly aware of the importance of their health and fitness. Most physicians and health care professionals encourage this movement, making a vital contribution to an healthier America.

Just by walking regularly, you induce your own internal mechanisms to prolong life and improve health. It may take several years to reach an absolute peak, but it can be done. Those who exercise throughout their lives have leaner bodies, stronger hearts, more efficient muscles, and are generally more productive overall than those who are sedentary. Without question they live longer and their normal physiologic aging processes are considerably slowed by exercise.

Make no mistake: Persistence is important. Exercise isn't like putting money in the bank, making deposits periodically and letting it accumulate interest. There is no shortcut to continuing the overall total fitness program on a daily basis. Pursuing fitness must become a way of life—to realize the benefits, you have to stick with it. Generally, once you get off to a good start, you feel so good you want to stay with the program for a lifetime. Like any other habit, once established, it becomes as easy as brushing your teeth.

How to Take Your Pulse

The easiest and simplest place is at your wrist, on the thumb side (the radial artery). Place the fingers of your other hand gently over the artery just one-half inch up your wrist from the base of the thumb. The pulse can be felt off to the side of the visible tendons that run down the center of your wrist's underside.

The second location is in the neck. Press your thumb and first finger (spread about an inch apart) on either side of your Adam's apple, just below your jaw. Don't press too hard, for this can slow your heart rate and you'll get an inaccurate reading. The third method is to press lightly with your fingers on your temple just in front of the upper part of your ear; the temporal artery can be felt here above the back tip of your jaw. Take a few practice readings when you are rested and relaxed. Take your pulse early in the morning before getting up to obtain a record of your resting pulse. You can closely estimate your heart rate by counting your pulse for ten seconds, multiply by six; fifteen seconds, multiply by four; or thirty seconds, multiply by two. In the majority of people, the resting pulse rate is between fifty and ninety beats a minute.

I suggest this experiment: Take your true "resting pulse" before you get out of bed in the morning. Then take your pulse just before you start your walk; then take your pulse the moment you have finished your walk. Finally, take your pulse three to five minutes after stopping walking. Your pulse rate will rise to its maximum at the end of the walk and will drop off close to the level it is during the day in three to five minutes after stopping. If you take your resting pulse rate each morning before rising, you will find it gradually drops, the fitter you become. Your heart is needing fewer beats to sustain you. While you have your watch out, you can also learn your rate of walking. If you take twenty minutes to walk one mile, you are walking at a rate of three miles per hour.

The Step Test

The step test is a proven method for measuring your heart's response to exercise. The step test can be done on a stool eight-inch height that allows you to step up and step down. It can also be done on any stairs of eight inches in height. Take two complete step-ups every five seconds, or twenty-four complete step-ups in sixty seconds. The duration for the test is three minutes. A complete step has four footfalls: Both feet step up one after the other, both feet return to the floor one after the other. The process is repeated to complete a "step-up." Say to yourself: "up, up, down, down, up, up, down, down" within a five-second span in order to establish the proper speed. To determine your heart rate recovery, start counting your pulse thirty seconds after your last step down and continue counting for thirty seconds until the one-minute post-exercise period. Count the total number of heart beats during this thirty-second period. This is your heart rate score. This rate will be about five times your resting pulse and is classified as light physical activity.

With increasing levels of overall fitness, the resting pulse decreases, as does your pulse all the time. The fitter you become, the more work is done with less effort.

The Best Exercise

The body generally prefers walking to other exercise. When I awake in the morning my body rebels against the idea of running (and I have been running now for fifteen years), yet it readily accepts a walk. Alternating walking and jogging is acceptable, but just walking is a more natural activity. We do it every day without thinking about it. Children start walking in the first year of life and become capable in no time.

All movement is good movement, but there is a minimum pace to get the desired results. Thornton Wilder once listed two hundred ways of saying a person was drunk. The number of words to describe a walk are also many: saunter, stroll, plod, step, stride, amble, pace, strut, stalk, tread, putter, prance, bounce, march, shuffle, mince. Any of these types, done long enough and frequently enough, will lead to fitness. An ideal walking pace is described as comfortable, but between "light" and "somewhat hard" is the level at which fitness follows. This corresponds with a "comfortable" pace of 50 to 60 percent of the predicted maximum heart rate. A good rule of thumb to determine your predicted maximum heart rate is to subtract your age from the number 220, then train (walk) at 50 to 60 percent of that heart rate.

Live Long, Die Fast

The breakthroughs of many of the world's great thinkers came to them while out for a walk. Ralph Waldo Emerson, American poet and essayist, frequently made notes while walking. The following is excerpted from a lecture he gave in 1858, published posthumously as "Country Live" in *The Atlantic* (November 1904):

Walking has the best value as gymnastics for the mind. "You shall never break down in a speech," said Sydney Smith, "on the day on which you have walked twelve miles."..."Walking," said Rousseau, "has something which animates and vivifies my ideas." And Plato said of exercise that "it would almost cure a guilty conscience."

Few men know how to take a walk. The qualifications are endurance, plain clothes, old shoes, an eye for Nature, good humor, vast curiosity, good speech, good silence, and nothing too much. If a man tells me that he has an intense love of Nature, I know, of course, that he has none. Good observers have the manners of trees and animals, their patient good sense, and if they add words 'tis only when words are better than silence. But a loud singer, or a storyteller, or a vain talker profanes the river and the forest, and is nothing like so good company as a dog.

When Nero advertised for a new luxury, a walk in the woods should have been offered. 'Tis one of the secrets for dodging old age. For Nature makes a like impression on age as on youth. Then I recommend it to people who are growing old against their will. A man in that predicament, if he stands before a mirror, or among young people, is made quite too sensible of the fact; but the forest awakens in him the same feeling it did when he was a boy, and he may draw a moral from the fact that 'tis the old trees that have all the beauty and grandeur.

I think 'tis the best of humanity that goes out to walk. In happy hours, I think all affairs may be wisely postponed for this walking. Can you hear what the morning says to you, and believe that? Can you bring home the summits of Wachusett, Greylock, and the New Hampshire hills? The Savin groves of Middlesex? The sedgy ripples of the old Colony ponds? The sunny shores of your own bay, and the low Indian hills of Rhode Island? The savageness of pine woods? Can you bottle the efflux of a June noon, and bring home the tops of Uncanoonuc? The landscape is vast, complete, alive. We step about, dibble and dot, and attempt in poor linear ways to hobble after those angelic radiations. The gulf between our seeing and our doing is a symbol of that between faith and experience.

No man is suddenly a good walker. Many men begin with good resolution, but they do not hold out, and I have sometimes thought it would be well to publish an Art of Walking, with Easy Lessons for Beginners. These we call apprentices. Those who persist from year to year, and obtain at last an intimacy with the country, and know all the good points within 10 miles, with the seasons for visiting each, know the lakes, the hills, where grapes, berries and nuts, where the rare plants are; where the best botanic ground; and where the noblest landscapes are seen, and are learning all the time—these we call professors.

Walking is often described by famous people as the best activity for inspired thought. In a book written in 1555, Cristobal Mendez made walking his first choice of exercise. He obtained the desired exercise by walking fast enough to make a slight acceleration of breathing, but he could still observe, read, or talk, whichever he chose. He felt he could practice his mental skills and philosophize on any topic while walking.

Because walking is so much more automatic than other actions, it requires almost no attention to safety or the outside world. You can dip into your mental and emotional worlds while walking.

Walk the Walk

Most people don't know that building and maintaining self-confidence involves how you carry yourself. How you walk and move influences how you think and feel. And self-confidence is the most important mental ingredient for success at anything.

In other words, learn how to walk the walk. Walking the walk involves holding your head high, with your chin up and eyes forward and focused. Shoulders are drawn back from your chest, arms swing, and you have a bounce in your step. If your body is up, your feelings and thoughts will be up.

If your body is down, your feelings and thoughts will be down. Features of not walking the walk include the head and eyes down, shoulders slouched, feet dragging with no energy in your step. It is very difficult to be walking the walk and saying things like "I'm awful, I can't do this, I am not worth much." Similarly, it's hard to be not walking the walk and saying things like "I am a great walker, or librarian, or carpenter; I am confident in my ability and I know how to handle pressure." This is because, in both cases, what you are saying to yourself is inconsistent with how you are carrying yourself.

Practice walking the walk by paying attention to how you carry yourself; focus on making positive physical changes when you walk. By walking the walk you will find that you naturally feel more positive and energetic.

Yes, walking is exercise; no, it is not too good to be true. Walking is not simply a trend—it will never be "out." It is a sound and sane option in a fitness-crazed world.

Part Three

Changes of Life

Old age, especially an honored old age, has so great an authority, that this is of more value than all the pleasures of youth.—Cicero

Chapter Eight

To Sleep, Perchance to Dream

To die, to sleep;
To sleep! Perchance to dream:
Ay, there's the rub.
For in that sleep of death what dreams may come?
—William Shakespeare

About one-third of a human lifetime is spent in sleep, yet we know relatively little about it. We usually think of sleep as a period of slowing down, of decreased activity. Actually, a lot of complex activity goes on in the brain and the body during sleep. The body's operating systems are not suppressed; in fact, some are more stimulated while asleep than awake. Even formulating a definition of sleep is not easy. And what controls this cyclic behavior, sleeping and waking, as night follows day?

How Much Sleep Do You Need?

The number of sleep hours people require varies widely. There is no "normal" amount; different people have different sleep needs. A "good night's sleep" ranges from less than three hours to more than ten. The average, of course, has been reported at eight hours, but seven to seven and a half is a more realistic estimate.

Humans, like all species, are different from one another. I don't wear the same size shoe that you do and you don't wear the same size your neighbor wears. Yet, for some strange reason, we are all expected to sleep the same amount of time. Don't worry if your sleep pattern doesn't conform to the magic eight-hour standard. Two people out of ten (slightly more in men) sleep less than six hours each night. One in ten sleeps nine hours or more a night. The long and short of it is, there are short sleepers and there are long sleepers, just as there are log sleepers and toss-and-turn sleepers.

The amount of sleep a certain individual needs remains constant, however. You may sleep longer one night than the next, depending on stress, emotions, and other life circumstances, but the hours you sleep over a week or a month average out to be about the same. One week generally falls within a half hour of the next.

A few people get along quite well on very little sleep—as little as two to three hours a night—and function as well as the rest of us. Napoleon and Edison were both short sleepers, about four to six hours a night. I know of one seventy-one-year-old woman who never slept more than three hours a night during her entire adult life. She felt quite well during the day. She cross-country skied every day in the winter, hiked frequently in the summer, and was a vigorous political activist. When she was studied at a sleep center at Dartmouth College, her sleep was found to be exceptionally sound, and overall, she was quite healthy.

A well-known physicist needed ten hours of sleep a night. With only eight hours, he was unable to concentrate, felt "foggy," and was unable to do his research. The person I'm talking about is Albert Einstein. He was a long sleeper, as are many creative people in science and the arts.

Interestingly enough, 150 years ago, before Thomas Edison invented the electric light bulb, Americans slept about an hour longer. Some researchers say it hasn't hurt us to stay up this extra hour; we just sleep a little more soundly and deeply.

> It is no small art to sleep—to achieve it one must stay awake all day!
>
> —Friedrich Wilhelm Nietzche

Does Your Sleep Change as You Age?

Sleep patterns do change later in life. As you age, you sleep more lightly. The quality of sleep usually diminishes, becoming lighter, less efficient, and less restful. "Delta" sleep, which is the deepest sleep and is associated with growth and bodily recovery, gradually decreases as you age. At about age fifty for men and sixty for women, there is measurably less delta sleep. Thus, older people are aroused easily by noise they slept through when they were younger.

In a healthy person, the length of time spent sleeping remains stable from about age twenty to seventy-five, but sleep problems increase. Sleep is more disturbed; thus, sleep time is lost because of inadvertent waking. Older people spend more time in bed and may think they sleep longer, but sleep is really interrupted by brief periods of wakefulness. Some older people experience hundreds of short awakenings at night. These short awakenings usually last fifteen seconds or less, but can leave the impression that one has been awake all night. I find that just knowing this helps me relax more during sleep.

What Happens during Sleep?

To understand mental activity during sleep, it is helpful to understand the normal functioning of the brain. As measured by an electroencephalogram (EEG), which records brain waves through electrodes placed all over the head, nerve cells in the brain fire individually. A brain wave is recorded as the average of millions of nerve cells as they fire. When awake, the positive and negative electrical charges of these nerve cells cancel each other out and the average approaches zero, resulting in a very small fluctuation from positive to negative. When asleep, more nerve cells work in synchrony and, like a lot of feet tapping to the same beat, they fire simultaneously, making the waves slower and larger. When awake, brain waves are small, fast waves, called alpha waves; when asleep, the waves are slower and bigger, called delta and theta waves.

There are two kinds of sleep: rapid eye movement (REM) sleep and non-REM sleep. During REM sleep, of course, the eyes move rapidly. During REM sleep is when dreaming occurs. We seem to look around in our dreams. This eye movement is visible simply by watching the closed eyelids: if the eyeball beneath the lids moves rapidly, the person is dreaming. Sometimes there are pauses between flurries of eye movement. Before the onset of a dream, a collection of nerve cells deep in the brainstem relaxes the muscles so deeply that they are nearly paralyzed. During a dream, however, the brain seems not to know that dreaming is taking place and gives commands to muscles to carry out the actions being dreamed about. These movements are rather limited, allowing us to sleep through our dreams.

People normally dream several times each night. In normal sleep, REM occurs every ninety minutes or so. The first REM period is very short, about five minutes. The second, ten minutes, and the third, twenty minutes. The final dream of the night lasts between thirty minutes and an hour.

The function of sleep, of course, is to rest the body and mind, to restore energy reserves. There are four stages in sleep. The first is a transition phase between waking and sleeping. Some parts of the brain are asleep; others are not. Stage 1 sleep is of little value in terms of bodily recovery. Stage 2 sleep, which is the most common sleep during the night, is a little deeper, and results in some rejuvenation. The sleep during Stages 3 and 4 is much deeper. Called delta sleep, Stage 3 and 4 sleep rejuvenates the body and restores energy, enthusiasm, and optimism. Hence, if we don't get enough delta sleep during the night, we may wake with a feeling of tiredness or malaise, even pessimism.

An interesting aspect of sleep concerns blood flow. During delta sleep, most of the blood is directed away from the brain toward the muscles. The brain can think during delta sleep, but it is sparse and fragmented, the result of too little blood. During REM sleep, when the brain partially wakes and thinking (dreaming) is more intense, more blood is flowing into the brain and less into the rest of the body. Some scientists estimate that a quarter of all the blood circulating during REM sleep is through the brain, presumably to support the increased brain activity of dreaming.

What If You Don't Get Enough Sleep?

The main consequence of a poor night's sleep, or even three or four nights of poor sleep, is simply sleepiness, and lost enthusiasm and motivation. Performance is not usually affected by losing one night's sleep, but judgment or creative thinking may be a little impaired. It is more difficult to focus attention, and reaction time is slowed. Monotonous activities, such as driving long distances, can be risky. After a sleepless night the majority of people will feel the most sleepy at about four or five o'clock in the morning, but then get a second wind around eight or ten and go on to function fairly well for the rest of the day.

Chronic sleep loss is a different story. Prolonged sleeplessness result in lapses of attention, slowed response, impaired thinking, strange and erratic behavior, and irritability. Mental functions fade, and judgment is impaired—enough to be dangerous.

In 1959, a disk jockey, Peter Tripp, went without sleep for 200 hours in a fund-raising effort for the March of Dimes. After five sleepless days, hallucinations occurred. At one point, he reportedly thought a tweed suit was made of worms, and saw flames coming out of a drawer. He was able to perform his day-time broadcast, but was frightened and thought he was in danger at night. At the end of his sleepless stint, he slept for thirteen hours straight. Outwardly, he seemed to recover quickly and appeared to be normal, but he reported depression for months afterward.

Many experiments have been conducted involving prolonged sleep deprivation, intentionally and unintentionally. Early on, mood deteriorates. Happiness and optimism disappear. People become sleepy and very groggy. In two or three days, "mini-sleeps" begin—lapses of attention when the brain goes to sleep for five to ten seconds and wakes immediately. After five days, these mini-sleeps become longer and more frequent. After ten days, subjects can't tell if they are awake or asleep. They talk, and in the middle of talking have two or three waves of sleep. They can walk, but may catch a few seconds of sleep from one step to the next. Mistakes are made trying to remember, focus, and respond to commands. Ultimately, they become depressed.

Many of us get less sleep than our bodies need. We accumulate sleep debts. Minor sleep losses built up over time are cumulative. Like unlucky gamblers, the sleep-deprived live perpetually "in the red," unable to perform their responsibilities at work, using drugs for temporary relief, and doing a progressively less efficient job. Such people should never be in positions of responsibility—flying an airplane or making decisions that affect others' health, for example.

The obvious conclusion here is to pay attention to your own sleep patterns. Learn what your body needs so you can recognize when you are suffering from sleep debt.

Are You an Insomniac?

Some people can't fall asleep, others can't stay asleep. The means of classifying insomnia vary: In one system, insomniacs are divided into people who can't fall asleep when they go to bed, and people who fall asleep readily, but can't stay asleep. The second system is based on how long the insomnia lasts: transient insomnia (one to three nights); short-term insomnia (three nights to three weeks); and chronic insomnia (more than three weeks). A third system classifies insomniacs according to the causes of their insomnia: (1) psychological problems; (2) medical problems; (3) lifestyle; and (4) poor sleep habits. Types 3 and 4 are far and away the most common and can be readily managed.

The Long and Short of Sleeping Pills and Sedatives

The search for sleep-inducing potions has preoccupied humanity for ages. Poppy syrup, belladonna berries, wild lettuces (Lattuca virosa), mandrake roots, and cowslip wine were used by primitive peoples. Phenobarbital, chloral hydrate, Flurazepan, and dihydrochloride are just modern versions of the kava-kava weeds. You'd think science would have made improvements over such folk medicines. Not so. There's very little difference between old and new sedatives. What most sedatives do, in effect, is obliterate consciousness. The ideal sedative, which sleep experts say should mimic the body's own sleep-producing chemistry, does not exist. Phenobarbital, for example, is a "knockout" drug; the insomniac who takes it does not sleep a natural, restful, repairing sleep. What's more, sleeping pills are addictive and can have consciousness-altering effects.

By and large, sleeping pills should be avoided. If you do take them, however, remember: Medications are metabolized and excreted more slowly as you age. What was once a proper dose may now result in an overdose.

Medicines Hazardous to Your Sleep

"Polypharmacy" is the practice of an individual taking three to ten or more drugs at the same time; often each drug has been prescribed by a different doctor. Such combinations may bring on insomnia. The following is a list of common insomnia-causing drugs:

- Antidepressant drugs, especially monoamine oxidase inhibitors
- Any drug with amphetamine, which is in prescription diet pills
- Drugs for high blood pressure
- Birth-control pills, although this is rare
- Broncho-dilating drugs (for asthma) containing ephedrine, aminophylline, or norepinephrine
- Caffeine-containing medications
- Sleeping pills and tranquilizers (insomnia can result from withdrawal on nights you do not use them)
- Steroid drugs, hormones, some thyroid preparations
- Some chemotherapeutic drugs for cancer
- Adrenocorticotropic hormone, or ACTH
- Dopa for Parkinsonism

Sundowners Syndrome

As the brain ages, some people require more stimulation to remain functional and rational. Some older people are oriented and function well during the day, but when night falls, stimulation decreases and they become agitated and confused. This is termed "Sundowners Syndrome."

What You Can Do

Assessing Your Own Insomnia

Self-evaluation procedures are a reasonable approach to insomnia, initially. If unsuccessful, consultation with a sleep specialist is in order. Sleep disorder centers and laboratories are prevalent in the United States; they can be found in forty of our fifty states and are usually associated with medical schools.

The first step in self-evaluation is to keep a sleep log and a day log. Depression, anxiety, and lifestyle sleep inhibitors are good things to watch for. A sleep history analysis, which is typically gleaned from a simple questionnaire, and a sleep hygiene analysis can also be useful. Other considerations: possible medical illnesses, overuse of medication, and characteristics of the bedroom, including the bed itself and the presence of light.

Self-evaluation is useful because it is empowering. It makes you believe, properly so, that you are in control, not helpless. Likewise, there are some easy steps you can take that may solve your insomnia altogether. At the very least, they can do no harm.

1. Reduce, preferably eliminate, your caffeine intake. Caffeine and similar stimulants cause health problems, particularly insomnia. Sensitivity to caffeine increases with age in many people. You may be exceptionally sensitive to this drug and unable to sleep after only one cup of tea or a chocolate bar. Caffeine continues to circulate in the blood after it is ingested, and may be excreted from your body more slowly than other drugs.

It's easy to ingest caffeine during the day. More than 300 milligrams of caffeine can be found in three cups of coffee or cola, certain pain tablets, a milk chocolate bar, or a dark chocolate bar. In addition, caffeine is addictive. In fact, people sensitive to caffeine can become addicted by consuming just one cup of coffee a day, or even one cola at lunch.

Virtually all soft drinks, unless specifically stipulated on the label, contain caffeine—from 15 milligrams per serving to as little as 1.2 milligrams in one diet cola. Most over-the-counter drugs also contain caffeine, including common non-prescription pain tablets, diuretics, and cold and allergy remedies. Virtually all weight-control aids contain large amounts of caffeine—200 milligrams or more in Dexatrim, Dexadiet, and Dietac. Similarly, alertness tablets, such as NoDoz and Vivarin, contain between 100 and 200 milligrams of caffeine.

Caffeine addiction is usually the last thing people think of as the cause of their insomnia. But addiction isn't the only problem with caffeine. High caffeine intake can lead to emotional behavior, tearfulness, lack of energy, depression, headaches, lethargy, irritability, and tension. Frequent urination during the night can also be caused by caffeine, along with urgency of urination in the daytime.

If you feel you must have caffeine in your life ("I can't do anything before I have my coffee"), don't kid yourself. You don't need it. There is nothing in the human body that requires caffeine to function. Be forewarned, however, getting off caffeine can be difficult, just like any other detoxification. Gradual reduction is usually recommended. To reduce caffeine, throw out the first cup of tea made from a tea bag and drink the second instead. Drink decaffeinated coffee, tea, and soft drinks. Read the labels on medications and buy those which do not contain caffeine. Remember to watch the chocolate.

2. Limit, preferably eliminate, alcohol. A popular prescription for insomnia is a cocktail or glass of wine at bedtime. This practice is ridiculous, plain and simple. In no way can alcohol be a sleeping aid. The sensation of deep relaxation that comes with alcohol is false. The truth is, sleep is compromised—normal sleep, that is. In fact, chronic alcoholics suffer from insomnia because the normal mechanisms of sleep simply cannot establish themselves.

3. Eliminate smoking. Smokers have greater difficulty falling asleep because cigarettes raise blood pressure, increase the heart rate, and stimulate brain activity, all of which compromise normal sleep mechanisms. Nicotine is a stimulant. Lighting a cigarette when you're unable to sleep at night will only perpetuate the problem. Pick up a book instead.

Other Solutions

- Napping: As we age, we tend to treat ourselves to naps during the day, making us even more wakeful at night. Denying yourself these naps may help you sleep through the night. Likewise, do not make a habit of turning over and going back to sleep in the morning. It may seem like a privilege of retirement, but if you are an insomniac, it will only exaggerate the problem. It is more difficult to fall asleep the next night and soon you will have initiated a vicious cycle. In addition, don't sit around all day doing nothing. You must have stimulation and activity during the day if you are to have a good sleep at night. Give yourself some reasons to need rest and sleep.

- Your bedroom: The environment where you sleep is important. Is the bedroom too hot? Too cold? Is the bedroom noisy? Is there a restless pet (dog, cat, or bird) scratching around at night? Is it too light or too dark? Are the windows readily opened or closed? How is the heating system? Does the furnace make noise that distracts you? What is the humidity? Dry air may lead to dry skin, a scratchy throat, and a stuffy nose. Excess humidity may cause sweating. If you have allergies, is pollen getting access to the bedroom?

   Many insomniacs dislike a noisy clock or a brightly illuminated digital clock staring them in the face all night. It creates a certain anxiety as they try to put off checking it for how many hours they have been awake. For other people a clock is reassuring, especially when they think they haven't been sleeping and discover three hours have passed.

- Your bed: Do you have a lumpy mattress? Is it sagging on the edges or the middle? Is it dusty? Maybe it's time to buy a new mattress or box spring. Maybe the bed isn't big enough, especially if there are two of you sleeping in it. Consider a king- or queen-size bed, or put twin beds side by side; you might sleep better. Is the pillow comfortable? Are the blankets too light? Heavy? Scratchy? Hot? Are the sheets fresh? Are they comfortable? Satin sheets may be sexy, but they may also be too slippery or block air flow. Likewise, muslin sheets may be too rough and flannel sheets too warm. Smooth cotton percale is perhaps the ideal.

On considering the purchase of a mattress or bed, spend some time thinking about basic mattress types: inner spring, foam, or water. Check on the firmness of the inner spring; the thicker the wire and the more turns in the spring, the firmer the mattress. If you buy a waterbed, be sure it is waveless, with built-in baffles, a liner, and a reliable, even heater.

There are special contoured pillows on the market that are worth considering. One I recommend is Wal-Pil-O, which supports the neck. A foam rubber slant is sometimes useful if you have problems with heartburn, breathing, or snoring. Many people sleep better if their head and upper trunk are elevated about six inches.

• Other considerations: Are your pajamas or nightgown comfortable? Do you need bed socks? Some people don't sleep well because they feel unsafe in bed. Consider installing a safer door, new locks, a smoke detector, a burglar alarm system, or whatever it takes.

Though I'm reluctant to bring it up, perhaps you should consider whether sleeping with someone is really best for you. In a study of couples who sleep together, some were asked to sleep together some nights and spend the others in separate beds. Researchers found that some people dreamed more when sleeping with their partner, resulting in less of the delta sleep needed for body recovery. At least ten minutes of deep, undisturbed sleep are necessary before deep delta sleep can develop. If one partner moves during those ten minutes and disturbs the other, the clock is apparently set back to zero and the ten minutes must start over again. Don't compromise marital bliss, certainly—I'm not suggesting that everyone sleep in separate beds. But if you are having trouble sleeping, at least consider it.

Along the same lines, do you and your partner go to bed at the same time? If one partner goes to bed two hours after the other, the disruption may compromise the other's sleep pattern. Reading at night with a light clipped to your book may disturb your partner less. Different things work for different people.

Exercise for Sleep

Fitness definitely facilitates healthy sleep patterns. Regular exercise, especially as you age, not only initiates sleepiness, it deepens your sleep to the delta level. Exercise should be part of any effort to reverse insomnia. You must tire your body if you hope to sleep well. Exercise also induces the release of endorphins, which naturally relieve depression and create a sense of well-being, which in turn restore a healthy sleep pattern.

Fitness also affects body temperature. The temperature of the human body normally goes up during the day and down at night, a built-in diurnal biological rhythm we all have. It peaks at mid-afternoon and is at its lowest around 5:00 a.m. These peaks and lows vary about two degrees (Fahrenheit) in young people, with less variation as you grow older. Insomniacs also have a narrower and shallower temperature rhythm than normal sleepers. Temperature increases less during the day because they are less alert and less active. This brings us back to exercise.

Increasing your body temperature five or six hours before going to bed induces a readiness to sleep. Any exercise will help you sleep if intensive enough to raise your core body temperature two degrees for at least twenty minutes. Over time, exercise can bring your temperature range back to the level you had when you were young. Changes in body temperature also explains the sleep-inducing effects of soaking in a hot tub, which can also be a viable method of treating insomnia.

Remember, though, the activity must be performed five or six hours before you want to sleep. If you are exercising at night, don't go at it hammer and tongs until 11:00 p.m. and expect to fall asleep at 11:15. The body needs to wind down before going to sleep.

Dietary Implications

Overall, you sleep better if you're healthy, and a major key to being healthy is diet. Diets lacking proper nutrients have been found to cause insomnia, and improving dietary intake has been shown to significantly help people with insomnia, especially those over forty. The following list of tips should start you in the right direction:

- Eat lots of salads and fresh vegetables. Avoid pre-packaged, pre-cooked, and chemical-filled foods, such as TV dinners. Fresh, unprocessed food is better for you.
- Buy vegetables fresh, store them for only a short time, and don't overcook them. Crunchy steamed vegetables have more vitamins than overcooked, soggy ones.
- Eat lots of whole grains and fiber foods. Instead of sugar, cake, pie, and white bread, consume complex carbohydrates: potatoes, pasta, fruits, salads, vegetables, whole-grain breads, and unsweetened cereal.
- Eat a variety of foods. Your body needs more than fifty nutrients for optimal health, and no single food contains all the essential nutrients.
- Limit fat. Avoid gravy, high-fat bread, and rich sauces. Eat less meat and more fish and poultry. Cut the fat off meat. Bake, broil, steam, roast, or stew; do not fry.
- Drink plenty of water—six to eight eight-ounce glasses

a day.

- Avoid snacks. Fatty foods, heavily garlic-flavored foods, or highly spiced foods are likely to give you indigestion or heartburn. In addition, many people are sensitive to monosodium glutamate (MSG), which can also cause insomnia. If you notice insomnia on nights you've eaten Chinese food, MSG may be the culprit. Remember, food allergies may cause insomnia, or a night eating habit (the Dagwood syndrome) may be at the root of the problem.

What's Going on in Your Head Is of Utmost Importance

The three biggest errors insomniacs can make are saying the following to themselves:

- "The longer I stay in bed, the more sleep I will get and the better I will feel." The longer you stay in bed, the worse you will sleep.
- "If I can't fall asleep, I simply have to try harder until I can do it." The worst thing you can do is try to sleep.
- "There's nothing worse than insomnia; it will ruin tomorrow and wreck my life." Whether you sleep or not probably won't make much difference in your performance. Famous insomniacs include Winston Churchill, Charles Dickens, James Thurber, Irving Berlin, Marilyn Monroe, Dorothy Kilgallen, Oscar Levant, and Napoleon Bonaparte.

The day will happen whether or not you get up.
—Source unknown

Relaxation Methods

The Bootzin Technique

Doctor Richard Bootzin, a sleep researcher, has worked out a technique, a type of stimulus-control therapy, designed to counteract conditioned insomnia:

1. Go to bed only when you are sleepy.

2. Use your bed only for sleeping. Do not read, watch TV, or eat in bed.

3. If you are unable to sleep, get up and move to another room. Stay up until you are really sleepy, then return to bed. If sleep does not come easily, get out of bed again. The goal is to associate the bed not with frustration and sleeplessness, but with falling asleep easily and quickly.

4. Repeat Step 3 as often as necessary through the night.

5. Set the alarm and get up at the same time every morning, regardless of how much or how little you slept during the night. This helps your body establish a diurnal rhythm.

6. Do not nap during the day.

Reducing tension and coping with stress are invaluable in correcting insomnia. Some people are able to relax easily, others are not. A number of relaxation techniques can diminish both psychological and musculoskeletal tension. Stretching before going to bed is often effective. Advanced relaxation techniques can also be helpful. Among these are biofeedback, meditation, autogenic training, progressive relaxation, so-called neurolinguistic programming, self-hypnosis, and hatha yoga.

Insomnia is an exasperating problem, affecting nearly every aspect of your life. Almost everyone suffers with it from time to time, but if it interrupts your life regularly, try some of the methods outlined above to overcome it—and seek help if it persists.

Chapter Nine

Sexuality: It Lasts as Long as You Do

So, lively brisk old fellow, don't let age get you down. White hairs or not, you can still be a lover.—Goethe

Old ladies take as much pleasure in love as do the young ones.
—Pierre de Bourdeille Brantome

Our society aggressively promotes youth: Never grow old, as they say. We are persuaded that sexual attractiveness is possible only with youthful bodies. For too many of us, the myths of aging—impotence, loss of sexuality, loss of sexual function, to name a few—become a self-fulfilling prophecy.

Dr. Alex Comfort distinguishes two kinds of aging: biological and sociogenic. Biological aging is manifest in such changes as graying hair, a decline in eye focusing power, a loss of hearing, and decreased elasticity in the skin (wrinkles). Sociogenic aging is the role society imposes on people once they reach a certain age. For example, the elderly in the United States are typically condemned as unemployable, unintelligent, senile, boring, set in their ways, expendable, and, last but not least, asexual.

It came as a great relief to me—as I hope it does to you—that these myths are utter nonsense. Sexuality and capacity for relationships normally last as long as you do. Contrary to popular opinion, sex after sixty is not the vice of the so-called dirty old man. Nor is it wishful thinking. While the intensity of sexual response does decrease, sexual interest, capacity, or activity does not have to cease at any age. Most elderly couples maintain a lively interest in sex, with only a gradual decline in frequency. Indeed, 75 to 80 percent report having sexual intercourse with considerable frequency. About 15 percent actually increase patterns of sexual interest and activity, probably the result of more privacy (children no longer at home), increased leisure time, and no fear of pregnancy.

According to a recent poll of women between the ages of forty and sixty-five, 89 percent consider themselves sexually appealing, 50 percent feel they are as appealing now as they were ten years ago, and 17 percent believe they are more appealing. What's more, 59 percent said they have sex as often or more often than when they were younger, and of the 95 percent who are finding their later years pleasurable, a rollicking 59 percent said they're experiencing the best years of their lives!

More good news: 94 percent consider a strong identity to be important to a high quality of living, and 53 percent ranked love as the most important thing in life while 97 percent ranked it very important. Of the 91 percent of respondents who are married, 70 percent said their marriages are very successful. And among the single respondents, 53 percent said they do not want to marry. Forty-eight percent were more attracted to older men than younger men. As women age, however, attraction to older men declines: only 30 percent of women between sixty and sixty-five find older men more appealing, the majority reporting that the appeal is energy and enthusiasm, as opposed to a younger body. The attitudes of these respondents debunk every myth about middle-aged and elderly women. The portrait that emerges is a promising one. These women are confident and relaxed. They enjoy life, and believe it's possible to get what they want out of it.

Despite evidence to the contrary, misinformation continues to surround maturing sexuality, particularly the fallacy that sexual desire automatically ebbs with age, primarily because personal information of this type can be so hard to obtain. Because of more conservative upbringing, today's older people feel a great deal of guilt about sexuality. Adhering to their conservative principles and strict religious mores, today's elderly tend to preclude divorce as an option; hence, many remain in marriages characterized by poor communication and little, if any, sexual activity. Even in their youth, today's older people were never as sexually active as the youth of today.

Older women, in particular, who show evident, even lusty, interest in sex are assumed to be suffering from emotional problems. Women who are obviously mentally stable and sexually active run the risk of being called depraved. Older men have it a bit better, but not much. What is lustiness in the young man is lechery in the old. Even simple affection can be misunderstood. An older man who shows warmth and affection toward children other than his own grandchildren or those of his friends, for example, runs the risk of having his motivation labeled sexual. (To set the record straight, child molesting, which is commonly associated with older men, is a crime committed primarily by men in their twenties.)

Even terminology shows prejudice: Old men become dirty old men. Old fools become old goats where sex is involved. Older women become biddies or hags. Biting humor implies impotence in older men and ugliness in older women. The expression "dirty old man" refers to a chauvinist to whom women are sexual objects or conquests, or both. And while we're on the subject of dirty old men, in my experience this archaic attitude toward women is not just exhibited by older men. Despite much progress by the women's movement, chauvinism abounds in men of all ages.

Yet another problem with getting accurate information about sexual activity among the elderly may be the conservative definitions used in questionnaires. Typically, what is considered sexual activity is strictly heterosexual and limited to complete intercourse. But such a narrow perspective is inaccurate and misleading. Contrary to popular myth, older homosexuals are no more lonely or unhappy than heterosexuals. In fact, one group of elderly homosexual men studied were found to exceed or equal comparable heterosexual groups on measures of life satisfaction. A full 75 percent were satisfied with their current sex life. Frequency of sexual activity remained stable, but there was a substantial reduction to fewer sexual partners over time. Homosexuals tend to be better prepared for coping with the adjustments of aging than heterosexual men and women, making such adjustments as planning for their own financial independence and deliberately creating a network of supportive friends.

Ironically, the taboo against inquiring into the sexuality of the elderly has become a self-perpetuating cycle. Older people are not asked about their sexual activity in surveys because everybody "knows" they aren't sexually active anymore. Because nobody asks, nobody learns otherwise; hence, the assumption is thought to be correct. Doctors contribute as well. Many do not ask their patients about sexual problems and functioning because they fear embarrassing them. By such an obvious omission, doctors perpetuate the embarrassment: Because older patients are not routinely asked, they are often ashamed to bring it up.

The societal standard that when you become old you become asexual has taken a physical toll, as well. Two disabilities now characterize sexual dysfunction in the aging: actual disease and the psychologically embedded belief inflicted by society. Decline in sexual vigor is attributable to any of the following: a general decline in physical and physiological capacity, boredom and overfamiliarity, illness, fatigue, preoccupation with other interests, loss of confidence in potency, high rates of overeating, and heavy use of alcohol. Why do these problems sound so familiar? Not one is unique to old age! Old people are simply people who have lived a long time. Both sexual desire and sexual capacity are lifelong. Even if intercourse is compromised by some major infirmity, other sexual needs persist: continuing closeness and sensuality, being valued as a man or woman, perpetuating self-esteem and self-worth.

Interest in sex remains relatively constant through life, it is true. However, there is a growing discrepancy between desire

---

There was Pantagruel, told by the keeper of the fountain that it was his wont to recast old women, so making them again young, and by his art to become like to the young wenches there present whom he had that very day recast—and altogether restored to that same beauty, form, size, elegance, and disposition of limbs and they had displayed at the age of fifteen or sixteen years, save only in regard to their heels, which were somewhat rounder than in their true youth. For this reason, from thence forth, upon meeting a man they were apter to fall on their backs. The band of old women attended upon the next round of recasting in great devotion and zeal, and importuned him on every hand, saying it was a thing in nature intolerable if a willing piece of tail lacked the looks to match. Pantagruel asking him by remelting and recasting old men, might likewise be remade, he answered that they could not, but that for them the manner of rejuvenation was by commerce with a woman renewed.

—Francois Rabalais

and practice. Yet another reason for reduced sexual activity in old age is lack of a suitable partner, particularly the death of a spouse. Because social contact between elderly men and women is often reduced, creating permanent and intimate connections is difficult, to say the least. In a study of sexual intercourse in elderly men, Weizman and Hart noted a decline in those between sixty-six and seventy-one years old, compared with men sixty to sixty-five, although the older group masturbated more often.

Clearly, this view of endless sex stands totally contrary to folklore. It defies society's views as well. But one thing is for certain: It is contrary to the attitudes and actions of nursing home administrators, many of whom disapprove of sexuality even among their junior staff, let alone their clients. As one article noted, "Nursing home operators seem to have sexual problems of their own. Otherwise it would be impossible to explain their attempt to run the nursing home as a mixed sex nunnery." Some directors do not allow married couples to share a room. Occasional "liberal" operators talk about providing petting rooms for inmates!

But what "inmates" here or anywhere else need is what is taken for granted by everyone else: privacy and the right to pursue relationships if they wish. What they do not want is a demeaning attempt to treat them as children. They do know their minds, and don't need their morals policed by busybodies who regard a normal sexual appetite in an older person as evidence of senility. According to one expert, "Old folks homes that adhere to the sexual mores of the outside world—instead of those of a boarding school—have happier and less deteriorated patients and a far lower consumption of drugs, especially tranquilizers." So ask before you sign yourself or your parent up; sexual policies are a good test of a nursing home's general recognition that those they house are people, not "cases" to be manipulated.

At any age, I recommend "living in sin" as a highly satisfactory alternative to loneliness. This is simply favoring sexuality with mutual support. Sometimes marriage compromises you financially, or you may have personal reasons for wanting to remain unmarried. The bottom line is, the nation, your state, your neighbors, and your children have no right to demand that you sign a marriage license. However, be informed of local and federal laws regarding your living arrangement. In the event of sudden widowhood, wives are entitled to security advantages, at least in states with community property laws.

Grown children can be a great trial to a parent in love. Children expect their surviving parent to show loyalty to the deceased parent by remaining single forever. They often actively discourage their parents from seeking new partners or behaving as sexual beings. Children traditionally do not look upon their parents as being sexual. They can't conceive of it being so. In this country especially, where there are already numerous hang-ups about the physical expression of a relationship, people don't like to think of their parents being involved in that way. They fear a change that is uncomfortable and, in their eyes, morally reprehensible.

Dr. Robert Butler, director of the National Institutes of Aging, thinks this may stem from uneasiness about what is going to happen to their own sexuality as they grow older. Other times children's discomfort results from a type of mental "enshrinement" of the deceased parent, Butler says. Children also worry that the parent (usually the mother) may end up being a caregiver, or may have to endure the pain of another loss. And not to be ignored is the worry about their inheritance, and whether the new love interest might interfere. Child interference can become quite extreme. Children can be irrationally critical and even try to obstruct the remarriage of their parents late in life. My advice: Just tell them you did your part raising them long ago, and press on with your own life. Do as you damn well please.

As we age, we retain a need for acceptance from society. But there is absolutely no reason for society's or a family's disapproval of marriage, even between parties of unequal age. Disapproval is more typically directed at the combination of a younger man and an older woman than the reverse, and it is often expressed as financial exploitation. Of course, you must not be naive about golddiggers, either. For example, a relationship of unequal age, regardless of the older partner's gender, may be improper if the older person loses his or her head, throwing caution to the wind and sacrificing sound judgment for the romance of it all. But remember, young people are permitted, even expected, to lose their heads when in love. Why, then, does society come down hard on "mature" people who do so?

Happily, some older people have a hardened resistance; in fact, many have enough common sense to just go on having sex without talking about it. These couples blissfully reject the images of the dirty old man and the nonsexual, undesirable older woman. This takes real bravery, bearing in mind that people in their eighties today were brought up learning sex education from the Victorians.

It's becoming easier and easier to find older couples meeting, falling in love, and living happily ever after. Older Americans are on the verge of making a sexual revolution of their own. If the kids don't like it, well, to hell with them. Really, it is none of their affair.

Competition

Sometimes there's no opportunity to maintain a sexually active life, despite an active interest in doing so. There are now, in the United States, about four unmarried women over the age of sixty-five for each unmarried man in the same age range. If all unmarried men over the age of sixty-five married women over the age of sixty-five, there would still be more than seven million women without husbands.

Women interested in a relationship are unlikely to find one easily, even if they overcome the hurdles posed by their children and society in general. Some women are simply too daunted by the competition and withdraw from the company of men. Women not feeling particularly beautiful, those who lack self-esteem, don't even try. Such women are often disdainful of men. "Humph," they will say. "They walk into the room, these men, and they sit around. They think they're the prize, and other women treat them as such." Not all women are interested in a relationship, however. Some women prefer intimate nonsexual friends to what they have always seen as a type of submission to a male.

On the other hand, faced with a four-to-one ratio, men may feel as though they're being attacked. This triggers their insecurity and prompts them to seek refuge with younger women. In nursing homes or retirement communities, some try to attach to younger female members on the staff, which usually ends up being a disappointment for both.

Homosexuality and masturbation are the only two options left open to the elderly without traditional partners. Even heterosexual activity is still only fully condoned with marriage. Many older people find it difficult to overcome their own prejudices, much less those imposed on them by their children or nursing home policies. Sadly, societal pressure eliminates these choices from consideration, even in our enlightened times.

Then there are individual sexual attitudes. Of the many studies I've reviewed, as well as the thousands of patients I have treated, I have seen a mix of people. Some had a high sexual drive; some had far less. There are those for whom sex is a principal resource, and those uninterested or embarrassed about it and therefore willing to lay it aside. There are people with no anxiety and very satisfying sex lives, and those with longstanding sexual disability. For folks happily active in youth, age does not abolish the need, the capacity, nor the satisfaction, unless illness negates their ability to enjoy sex or deprives them of a partner. In fact, those who rated sexual urges as strongest in youth rated them as moderate in old age, and most who described sexual feelings as weak to moderate in youth described themselves as without sexual feelings in old age.

People may elect to stop being sexually active because they want to, because they don't get much satisfaction from it, or because they are sick. It's all in the attitude. For some people, age can serve as a good, proper, and valid excuse for dropping a worrisome function. In otherwise happily married couples, when the normal level of sexual performance falls off, it is almost always accounted for by the illness of one spouse.

To enlighten the uninitiated, the study of sexuality isn't just genital stimulation. It encompasses the entire field of human contact. Communication is very much a part of it. Sexuality is the way people define and present themselves. Sexual expression enormously enhances self-esteem, self-worth, and self-image. Maintaining sexuality as you age requires an appreciation of sex as an expression of self, not a phase of the self used up in youth. It's a pity to be psyched out of something you value, especially by anxiety and wrong information. At age sixty-one, Ralph Waldo Emerson wrote in his journal, "Within I do not find wrinkles or a used up heart, but unspent youth!" We must enhance and intensify the quality of sexuality in old age by conveying a humanistic, pleasure-oriented point of view. Sexuality is an aspect of all chronologic ages and all states of health. It does not just go away.

I promote a view of sexual expression as an enriching experience that opens communication, increases intimacy, and bolsters self-esteem. Adopting this definition goes a long way to promote sexual adjustment as you age. It provides welcome reassurance against society's false expectations and hostility toward sexual matters. Despite the sometimes physical limitations of old age, people in their golden years usually have considerable free time, coupled with extensive life experience. What a sizzling combination! What better formula to bring to sexual expression? Don't let aging be a cold winter with no refuge—make it the harvest of a lifetime, the harvest of learning and loving.

As you age there can be less emphasis on the goal—namely, orgasm. Mature sex consists of more pleasuring, cuddling, touching, lovemaking nearly continually, with intercourse interspersed. As the measure of sexual expression, an age-related philosophy defines the quality of sexual experience over quantity. A heartwarming and inspiring story from one elderly pair says it well: "We take baths together. He washes my body, and I wash his. I know I'm getting old and my skin could use an ironing, but we love each other, so sex is beautiful."

Skilled and tender lovers, who take care of their personal experience, never stop augmenting their sexuality. They make up in proficiency and familiarity anything they may lack in looks. Sexual attractiveness has little to do with age, and the appearance of a partner is no index of sexual competence and skill (and good sex does require competence and skill!). Listen to this enviable "old" woman: "Sex isn't as powerful a need as when you're young, but the whole feeling is there: it's as nice as it ever was! He puts his arms around me, kisses me and it comes to me, satisfaction and orgasm, just like it always did. Don't let anybody tell you different. Maybe it only happens once every ten days to two weeks, but as you get older, it's such a release from tensions, even more than when I was young. I'm an old dog who's even learned a few new tricks—like oral sex, for instance."

Here is another mature notion of sex: "Sexuality is much more than genitalia; more than orgasm and it is more than any other physical means of stimulation. It is by all means the total human being who is involved emotionally, cognitively (intellectually), as well as physically."

In any relationship, young or old, those who focus on pleasing each other or on enjoying the other person, rather than aiming at the goalpost of orgasm, will have a much better relationship emotionally as well as physically.

With increasing age, traditional sexual roles are blurred. People no longer have to perform gender-specific tasks (home-making for women, breadwinning for men); their opposite gender characteristics are allowed to emerge. Older men exhibit more nurturing, and older women become more assertive. Older women get upset with older men who seem passive, because they think they're not supposed to be. The reverse is also true: Older men are put off by women who seem too dominant to be feminine. The breakdown of traditional roles is a good thing: More equality is often found in relationships between older people, and even more mutual satisfaction than may be present in younger couples.

The women's movement is a major force in the overt sexual awakening of the older woman. Women today enjoy a new assertiveness after forty. To quote one older woman: "Now when I'm in the mood, I wake him up. Afterward, I roll over and sometimes fall back asleep. He's been doing that to me for years!" These role changes for both men and women open the door to a whole new frontier, which can keep even a long-standing relationship perpetually changing in sexual expression.

What Sexual Changes Happen as You Age?

A general slowing of the human body occurs with age. We can make it less so with exercise, a positive attitude, and continued work and activity—all the things a person uses to maintain physical and emotional health—but the sexual response cycle does gradually diminish. The trick is to make it diminish as slowly as possible.

Some general effects of aging on sex are listed below.

Men

- There is a gradual decrease in circulating testosterone (male sex hormone).

- Penile erection takes more time, and it may not be as hard as earlier in life. Full turgidity and girth may be achieved only seconds before ejaculation. Direct penile stimulation is required more frequently.
- Nipple erection is less obvious.
- Ejaculatory control increases.
- Ejaculation may take place every time, or every second or third sexual episode. Ironically, more success is found if there's little preoccupation with orgasm.
- Sex flush is rare in men after fifty. (This resembles a "big blush.")
- Ejaculation is less powerful, and orgasm (though often only slightly) less intense. The ejaculate is expelled with slightly less force and contains less seminal fluid.
- Fertility levels are reduced, but men do not become sterile at any age.
- The refractory period between ejaculations becomes longer.
- Climax continues to provide extreme pleasure—it is still the most fun you can have without laughing!

Women

- Vaginal lubrication requires more stimulation.
- Expansion of the vaginal barrel in length and width is reduced.
- The lining of the vagina thins, and is therefore more easily irritated.
- The bladder and urethra may become irritated during intercourse.
- The clitoral size decreases and clitoral hood atrophies, as does the fat pad over the mons veneris (pubis).
- The orgasmic phase is shorter.
- The capability of multiple orgasms remains.
- Despite the hormonal reduction during menopause,

maintaining an active sex life can help retain vaginal lubrication capacity and regular contractions during intercourse. Contact with the penis helps preserve the shape and size of the vaginal space.

What You Can Do

What can you do to preserve your sexuality? First and foremost, simply recognize that, if cultivated, sexuality is lifelong in both sexes. If a problem with sex does arise, ferret out the cause and eradicate it. Whatever you do, don't assume it is the result of aging—it's not. Also, don't underestimate the power of sexual dysfunction. It can initiate such serious clinical symptoms as anxiety, depression, tension, and lowered self-esteem.

The ludicrous point is often made that sex can be dangerous for someone with heart disease or other problems. In truth, unwillingly ceasing sex is far more dangerous to someone's health than any associated exertion. In fact, stopping sex often leads to severe depression. Abstinence because of coronary artery disease or a major illness need only be limited to the time when you must avoid even minimal activity, like walking around the room.

What about Impotence?

Impotence in men is unrelated to age. It is often caused by performance anxiety, which is usually rooted in the belief that age compromises sexuality. About half of all men with severe diabetes become impotent; still, there are solutions even for them. For starters, medication and alcohol can compromise sexual functioning in many diabetics and hypertensive people. If you suddenly lose libido or potency while taking pills, don't be coy. Be forthright about sexual side effects when you see your doctor—he or she cannot spot them by extrasensory perception.

It has been rumored that problems with the prostate gland can also affect sexual functioning. The prostate gland, which is situated in the crotch, is sort of wrapped around the urethra (the tube proceeding from the bladder to the penis and to the outside), and gradually enlarges with age, although why this enlargement takes place is not entirely clear. Sexual sensations without orgasm have been said, by the uninformed, to aggravate it and sexual activity to prevent it. But no reliable data support this theory, either. Enlargement of the prostate gland may cause some pinching of the outflow of urine from the bladder, resulting in sensations of urgency, frequency, and difficulty in urination.

An operation called transurethral resection is a common cure. It is safe and can be done on healthy men at any age. When done conservatively, the operation removes nothing but the excessive prostate gland surrounding the urethra. This operation is necessary if disruptive urinary symptoms emerge—it's not going to just go away. Removing the prostate by this method does not affect sexual potency, but it may alter the sensation of ejaculation (sometimes, though rarely, the sensation is abolished). Untreated, however, an enlarged prostate can risk severe consequences to the waterworks and jeopardize potency.

More radical prostate operations cut the nerves controlling penile hydraulics. This procedure does result in impotence: Don't let anyone just do that to you! Discuss how the operation is done, and all its consequences. Determine precisely what the surgeon is going to do and why. Find out the expected result, in terms of both sexuality and urinary flow. Surgeons who value their own sexuality will, you can bet your bottom dollar, do everything they can to preserve yours. Lay it clearly on the line, just in case the surgeon upholds the myth that you should be sexually retired. (This attitude among surgeons is all too common.)

Most removed prostate tissue contains areas that look like cancer. They are usually not cancerous, however, and seem to do no harm. Real prostate cancer requires surgery and hormonal treatment. Management is really quite good, prostate cancer being one of the easiest cancers to treat successfully. Spread of the cancer to other organs can be controlled in most cases by using female hormones. This does turn off libido, but it may be a choice you have to make; spread of prostate cancer to bone can be painful and disabling.

The bottom line: Prostatic surgery should not impair potency if it is done well. I once heard an annoyingly ignorant, young urologist say that he prefers to do radical prostatectomies on older men because "after fifty, they won't need any sex anyway." In truth, half the men who give up sex because they're "too old" aren't impotent at all. And of the other half, those who are impotent, 90 percent have absolutely nothing wrong with their hydraulics—in other words, they can still have sex.

There is one real threat to sexuality that comes with aging: If sexual activity is stopped for any length of time, many have difficulty regaining sexual function. Often treatment is required to jump-start sexual function again. The best example of this is the widower whose wife dies after a long illness. He wants to remarry, but living the interim without sex, or having sex with a strange partner, even the natural guilt that results from feeling relieved at his wife's passing, can result in difficulty getting and maintaining an erection. But this type of impotency is totally reversible with time.

Women have the advantage of a longer life span and less coronary artery disease than men; hence the present ratio of widows to widowers. (If women continue to smoke cigarettes at the present rate, however, this advantage will diminish.) This ratio helps explain why men are often able to attract younger partners. Older women are subject to a sexual boycott by society. I don't have a good remedy for this. Though masturbation is an important and useful sexual response for both sexes at all ages, it is not a substitute for being sexually valued. The following are some things men and women can do to maintain their sexuality in their later years:

- Avoid obesity. It is not only unattractive by our social dictates, but interferes physiologically with erection. Cosmetic surgery may help as well—for example, immense pendulous breasts that get sore can be reduced through breast reduction surgery. This is not denying age, it's restoring function to the age you really are. Attractiveness is the visible indication of self-esteem. Use any means to stay active and avoid sloppiness of personal hygiene at any age.

- Avoid people you don't like, those who harp on your insecurities or tell you all about their fears of sex. Choose your direction according to who you are as a person, not how you look. A sexually capable man or woman who wishes to have sex with someone of the same age experiences him- or herself as a fully sexual person.

- Work with the minor effects of aging, not against them. Erection in aging men does differ from that of muscular youth in the amount and type of stimulation needed to produce it. After the age of fifty, for example, so-called psychic erection becomes less frequent, except in sleep, when it occurs just as often as in youth. A psychic erection results from just thinking about sex or seeing something sexual. Erection after age fifty may require two or three minutes of direct stimulation by rubbing or otherwise caressing. Both men and women should know this.

- Follow the rules of comfort: Don't worry, don't hurry. In fact, continue the preliminary stimulation until the gear, like a nosewheel, locks in position. Not "holding" an erection is caused by starting intercourse too soon or sudden changes in function (excluding causes

161

mentioned). If you ever get an erection on waking in the morning, in sleep, or during masturbation, it is a sure sign that nothing is wrong with the hydraulics!

- Keep a mature attitude. Far and away the most frequent cause of sexual nonfunction at all ages is performance anxiety. Don't treat sex as a performance. Firm erection can be produced by putting finger pressure just behind the scrotum, crossing the legs, or placing a tight band around the base of both the penis and scrotum. There's no magic here. But keep in mind, these methods are for people in a hurry. Adequate early handwork, without haste, grants both partners a far more rewarding sexual encounter.

- Males of all ages have unexplained periods of "running out of steam," as many put it. If you don't get paranoid about it, at most it lasts four or five days. Ill-advised boys and men who are obsessed with performance look on such events as the dreaded "beginning of the end." But be assured, it is only temporary. More competent and experienced lovers just switch techniques and enjoy the variety during this period. Many women make similar adjustments when they're menstruating, using the time to experiment with other forms of sex play.

- The "use it or lose it" and "rest and rust" admonition has an important role in sexuality. The few age-related genital changes there are (decreased lubrication, inelastic and thin vaginal tissues) are much less frequent in women who are sexually active, whether by masturbation or intercourse. Like it is for men, it usually requires several weeks or months for women to comfortably engage in sexual intercourse after an extended period of abstinence.

How about Hormone Therapy?

Very few men are deficient in testosterone. A drug called Mesterolone (Proviron), a synthetic hormone, may lower the stimulation threshold. This drug, though rarely useful, may "prime the pump." Its only advantage is that it does not cause your own central control mechanism to turn off internal hormone production, as taking testosterone does.

Female hormone replacement therapy is usually considered helpful, but about as often it is only cosmetic. For example, therapy has proven effective in keeping the vagina in good health, but frequent sexual activity has been found to be almost as effective, and much more gratifying. Hysterectomy or other pelvic surgery in women usually does not interfere with sexuality at all. And if the procedure is to repair sagging vaginal walls, it can vastly improve sensation for both partners.

Your doctor can help with the decision to use or not use estrogen replacement therapy. It certainly has a role: the genital lining (epithelium) may atrophy, causing vaginitis with irritation, burning, itching, vaginal discharge, dyspareunia (painful intercourse), and occasionally vaginal bleeding. Because the health of the membrane lining depends on estrogen, such symptoms of irritation as burning and painful urination may be helped with estrogen replacement.

> No spring nor summer beauty hath such grace as I have seen in one autumnal face.
>
> —John Donne

Did You Say Masturbate?

Masturbation used to be a focus of enormous medical, scientific, and moral fabrication. As I was growing up, masturbation had a terrible cloud of disapproval surrounding it, particularly by religious people. I remember being told that if you masturbated, you would lose your mind, or you would never be able to love anyone truly. What a lot of hogwash!

A sensible and even remotely biologically educated person knows masturbation is a normal, healthy act for any person, at any age, at any time. It is an integral part of human sexual behavior. In fact, its uses change throughout life. Preadolescent and adolescent masturbation is our most common path to sexual sensation. Later, masturbation becomes a sexual exercise, improving women's response and men's staying power. It even develops rings of fantasy.

In adult married life, masturbation is an integral part of love play and can be a source of variety. Mutual masturbation or individual masturbation of one's partner broadens sexual experience. In later life, it can be a good substitute for those without partners, or serve as a gentler source of orgasm for the ill. Masturbation has always been used as maintenance, a sexual outlet during periods without sexual activity. This is particularly important for men, who are more likely to find "restarting" hard to do and require a jump start.

With increasing age, males require manual stimulation to achieve firm erection. Don't be self-conscious about handwork on each other. As you age you may only achieve orgasm once in two or three acts of intercourse. The choice may become either you or your partner reaching climax manually. A word of warning: Using masturbation every time will raise the firing threshold, resulting in far fewer coital orgasms.

Women who learn to masturbate add it to their sexual program and use it throughout life when they wish. I've known women of seventy and eighty who had never had an orgasm— until they learned to masturbate. In a few instances, this occurred at the prompting of their daughters. Some were taught at a counseling clinic, having gone to the clinic because they didn't want to die without experiencing that part of their sexuality and womanhood.

I don't want to press any sexual activity on people who don't want it or who take it as an affront. However, masturbation is worth mentioning and it's never too late to buy stock in your own sexuality! Look on masturbation in later life as it is described: It is not a reversion, and God forbid that you think of it as a perversion. Masturbation is a healthy gesture of life-affirming defiance, a useful source of sexual pleasure that the antisexual people of the world can't keep you from enjoying. If you, as I, learned it in childhood, laden with guilt, and had two minds about it as an adult, reconsider it as an option in your golden years. Explore your own body leisurely, gradually, happily, comfortably, profitably, and do it now.

What about Fertility as You Age?

We used to say that female fertility ends at menopause. Have you read the papers lately? On record is a woman from Los Angeles who reportedly delivered a daughter at the age of fifty-seven! Postmenopausal women have been brought to successful completion of pregnancies—the brave new fertility world. A word of warning, however: If you are on the pill or some other hormone regimen, and you are not sure whether you have stopped ovulating, you could, on stopping the pill, get a surprise pregnancy. This is far from ideal if you don't need a baby in your old age, but more seriously, the risk of Down's Syndrome in the fetus increases with a mother's age.

Men retain lifelong fertility, even extending into their nineties and beyond. A sperm examination can settle this one way or another. It is the biological mechanisms that differ. Sperm are short-lived and made continuously, whereas all the ova a woman will ever have are present when she is born.

Unlike motherhood, fatherhood never becomes physically

risky. In fact, there is no scientific evidence that children of old fathers have any greater health risk than those of young fathers. With this gift of eternal fertility comes a responsibility, however. If you have a fertile partner and do not want children, don't let age make you careless about contraception. You may not be around for the whole period of fathering. Considering you'll probably need a run of at least sixteen years to see the job through, this rules out responsible procreation after the age of seventy.

Vasectomy is a good solution for men in their later years. Potency is not affected. On the contrary, the procedure was formerly done under the name of "Steinach's Operation" as a rejuvenating procedure. Although there is not much evidence that it rejuvenates, it does no harm. In fact, it brings welcome relief and freedom of expression to the female partner.

Sexuality with Illness and Disease

Arthritis

About 30 percent of people over the age of sixty-five are limited by some form of arthritis. This should not compromise sexual behavior, however. The following are practical suggestions for managing arthritis and maintaining sexual activity:

- Begin an exercise program to increase joint mobility.
- Do a series of stretches before sex, even incorporate them into foreplay.
- Use heat in a variety of ways to ease joints and increase mobility.
- Communicate with your partner about feelings of unattractiveness.
- Communicate about physical limitations. Avoid positions that put prolonged pressure on joints; experiment with adaptive positions.
- Learn alternatives to intercourse, such as mutual masturbation or oral sex.

- Use a waterbed.
- Place a pillow under painful limbs.

Cancer

As the leading cause of death in the United States, cancer elicits fear and horror, severe depression, and anxiety. But it doesn't have to limit sexual activity. Suggestions for maintaining sexual activity are as follows:

- Time your sexual activity around the pain, or medication schedule.
- Take a less active role.
- Use non-weight-bearing positions to avoid fatigue.
- Communicate with your partner about self-consciousness—operative scars, mastectomy, and so forth.
- Incorporate massage or deep breathing into your sexual activity.
- Reassure your partner that he or she is still sexually attractive and desirable.

Heart Disease

Coronary attacks prompt many people to give up sex altogether, fearing it will endanger their lives. This does not have to be. Suggestions for maintaining sexual activity following heart trouble include the following:

- Realize that the likelihood of heart attack during sex is very small.
- Increase time spent in foreplay to allow the heart to warm up gradually.
- Use energy-conserving, non-weight-bearing sexual positions.
- Improve overall fitness and endurance through an exercise program.
- Avoid sex when anxious or fatigued.
- Decrease performance anxiety.
- Masturbate.

Stroke (Cerebrovascular Accident, or CVA)

Hardly an uncommon ailment, there are 500,000 stroke victims each year; more than 200,000 survivors are added to the stroke population annually. Here, too, surviving a stroke does not mean you have to give up sexual activity. The following are suggestions for maintaining sexual activity for stroke victims:

- Use nonverbal communication to emphasize stimulation of areas still sensitive to touch.
- Use a waterbed.
- Explore through touch and smell, rather than depending on vision.
- Use a vibrator if hands are weak or uncoordinated.
- Share fantasies in writing.

Diabetes

Common in later life, many diabetic men are not truly impotent. However, it's one of the few illnesses that can cause chronic impotence by compromising the physiological mechanisms. The following are some suggestions for diabetic men to maintain sexual activity:

- Reduce anxiety.
- Communicate through touch, smell, and imagination. Share fantasies.
- Ask your partner to emphasize stimulation of areas that are still sensitive.
- Use a hard, donut-shaped rubber device slipped over the partially erect penis. It is helpful in maintaining an erection, and is available in shops that carry sexual aids. (Although rubber bands are sometimes used to accomplish the same effect, this is not recommended.)
- Seek counseling if impotence is psychogenic.

Sex and Drug Use

Here's an eye-opening statistic: The elderly make up 12 percent of the population but consume 30 percent of all prescription drugs. Usually they are not informed about the sexual implications associated with certain prescription drugs because of doctors' and pharmacists' presumption that old people are asexual. Many common drugs interfere with sexual function: antihistamines, barbiturates, librium, Thorazine, Tagamet, atromid, catapres, danocryne, Valium, antabuse, estrogen, licorice, steroid hormones, indural, Serpasil, aldactone, alcohol, anticholinergic, digitalis, norpace, penicillamine, phenothiazine, testosterone, Aureomycin, and diethylstilbestrol. Ask your doctor about possible side effects when he or she prescribes any medication. If the drug affects sexual functioning, request an alternative.

Sex and Your Doctor

Older Americans applaud the new openness about sex and romance for their generation. But physicians must catch up. They must recognize our changing sexuality as we age. Sexual dysfunction in older age is not caused by age but by specific, usually treatable, diseases or medication. Defend your sexuality against both failure to perform and unwise treatment and advice. Find a doctor with whom you can discuss sex, and who recognizes that sexuality at your age (and older) is normal.

I never dismissed it lightly when an older patient came to me with a sexual problem. Managing sexual problems in older people was one of the most satisfying aspects of my many years in practice. I enjoyed teaching both men and women the knowledge of normal physiologic changes associated with aging. Oftentimes this information greatly enhanced their adjustment toward and enjoyment of sexual expression.

Groups of older people, finally given leave by an uncritical listener or peers with the same feelings, often become candid about their sexual feelings and liberal in their sexual views. Generally, women experiencing sexual dysfunction because of loss of female hormone like to discuss the advisability of estrogen with their doctors. An elderly couple, once made aware of the tendency for an older man not to ejaculate every time he has sex, relaxes and enjoys the advantage of more frequent erections. They take advantage of the decreased recovery periods that result from less frequent ejaculation.

Sex and Romance

It occurs to me that romance for its own sake is becoming more and more scarce. Perhaps the energy and creativity for romance is being lost with the aging of a generation. Sexuality grows with experience. The romance of older people is very tender, very sensitive. It may be physical, it may include intercourse, or it may not. I suspect the old could probably show the young a thing or two about romance—dancing, walking hand in hand, candlelight dinners, for instance. And if our culture were more tolerant about love and sex among the elderly, the young would probably be able to learn it.

I think Jerome J. Goldstein said it best:

We are probably the only members of society in the history of mankind for which the younger generation has so little respect and has demonstrated such a shameful lack of regard. Senior citizens are constantly being criticized, belittled and sniped at for every conceivable deficiency of the modern world, real or imaginary. Upon reflection, I would like to point out that it wasn't senior citizens who took the melody out of music, or the beauty out of art, or the pride out of appearance, or the romance out of love, the commitment out of marriage, the responsibility out of parenthood, the togetherness out of family, the learning out of education, the loyalty out of Americanism, the service out of patriotism, the hearth out of the home, the civility out of behavior, the refinement out of language, the dedication out of employment, the prudence out of spending, or the ambition out of achievement. And we are certainly not the ones who eliminated patience and tolerance out of relationships.

Chapter Ten

Menopause: The Pause That Refreshes

Menopause—or "the change of life," as it is commonly called (I've always found this amusing, as if the rest of life held no changes!)—refers to the process that precedes the end of a woman's reproductive life. That's all it is, but like most bodily changes, menopause prompts apprehension in many women.

Technically, menopause lasts for just a week: the week of a woman's final menstrual period. The term climacteric covers the years surrounding menopause, which typically extend from the early forties to the early sixties, when production of estrogen gradually tapers off and ultimately stops altogether. That's when the ovaries retire, so to speak. Surgical menopause, of course, occurs when the ovaries are removed.

From the 1970s to the mid-1980s, relatively little was published about menopause. Too often, doctors didn't know as much as their patients did on the subject. But between 1985 and 1995, baby boomers entering midlife started demanding, and succeeded in getting, more attention and research devoted to menopause. Some say menopause has become positively chic today, studied by everyone from physicians to sociologists, from health activists to psychiatrists, from TV talk show hosts to best-selling authors. This trend is evidenced by a procession of somber articles in medical journals.

Of course, the focus on menopause has germinated as many questions as answers: Is menopause the end of youthfulness? Is it the threshold of what author Gail Sheehy calls a second adulthood? Is it a simple rite of passage or a minor biological event? Is it the onset of aging, wrinkles, and expanding waistlines? Is it the reflection of reduced synthesis in hormones?

Janine Cobb, at age sixty, came up with the idea of sharing information about menopause through a newsletter. Hundreds of women responded favorably. In 1984, she began publishing *A Friend Indeed;* today the subscriber base totals 6,000. Clearly, women want to learn more about "the change."

Hard-Wired Facts in the Biology of Reproduction

A human female fetus in the uterus at four months' gestation has two million (yes, you heard me correctly, two million) eggs, capable of developing and being fertilized to become a baby. By age fourteen, around the onset of the first menstrual period, about 400,000 eggs are left in the ovaries. By age forty, this figure has been reduced to 200,000, and they gradually fall in number. When the last egg induces the last menstrual period, menopause is over. No more eggs, no more babies!

A normal ovarian cycle lasts about twenty-eight days. Of the 400,000 eggs, one becomes dominant and grows. On the fourteenth day, the brain's pituitary gland secretes hormones that release that egg from the ovary. A structure called the corpus luteum, left behind by the egg, secretes estrogen and progesterone. These hormones prepare the uterus for implantation of the egg, in the event that it is fertilized by a sperm. How long the egg is capable of being fertilized is uncertain, but probably no more than about twelve hours after it is released from the ovary. On the twenty-second day, the corpus luteum begins to regress, and regression continues if the egg is not fertilized. The prepared lining of the uterus breaks down and is sloughed; bleeding and discharge through the vagina occurs as menstrual flow, which lasts from three to seven days. As women age, the number of eggs declines as they become less responsive to hormones from the pituitary gland. Cessation of fertility, or menopause, is a consequence of the ovaries not releasing any eggs.

Estrogen Therapy: To Be or Not to Be?

Until the 1960s, women regarded menopause as yet another natural passage. It was often quite troublesome, sometimes fearsome, but seldom did it require medical intervention. Then scientists learned how to synthesize and manufacture the hormones estrogen and progesterone. At that time, an unprecedented event occurred: The normal function of menopause was classified as a disease. Doctors extended the boundaries of their profession to include the definition and management of menopause. Gynecologists and obstetricians began prescribing estrogen therapy for practically all menopausal women for an indefinite period. Even medical textbooks commenced defining menopause as a disease deficiency, like diabetes.

In 1966, Robert Wilson published *Feminine Forever*. His crusade for estrogen replacement from menopause to the grave was funded by (surprise, surprise) the pharmaceutical companies that produced the drug. Wilson urged women to take estrogen and progesterone for menopause, warning, "no woman can be sure of escaping the horror of this living decay." Before long, estrogen had become one of the most popular drugs in the United States: six million women were taking it to "prevent aging."

To my knowledge, only one person, Kathleen MacPherson, professor and dean at the University of Southern Maine's School of Nursing, had the courage to challenge Robert Wilson. She was quoted as saying, "Wilson was widely dismissed as a quack by his more sober colleagues, but rarely in public and always off the record." Betty Friedan describes the estrogen therapy phenomenon in her book *The Fountain of Age:* "The overriding cause of this menopause mania is, of course, the sheer size of the market. Responsible health reporters have warned that the new breed of menopause mavens have personally profited from the expanding menopause market."

Then a cloud cast its shadow on the estrogen therapy parade. In 1975, a number of scientific studies uncovered an increased risk of uterine cancer in women who took estrogen replacement therapy. As a result, estrogen prescriptions decreased 40 percent. Not so easily deterred, pharmaceutical companies have responded by racing to develop safer, more acceptable hormone regimens. They aspire to capture a market that exceeds half a billion dollars, and continues to grow. If trends continue, upwards of 90 percent of women will take replacement hormones for three to five decades—well over a third of their lives.

The Good News

In the past, menopause was a taboo subject, seldom discussed or studied. It was generally regarded as the end of a woman's reproductive years, and was thought to be accompanied by depression. While some called menstruation "the curse," "falling off the roof," or "the scary nuisance," more irreproachable terms were reserved for menopause, including "the bleak event" and "the death of womanhood."

Victorian women assumed they could expect everything from shingles to insanity during "the change." Women were said to become peevish, irritable, morose, and depressed, an attitude implying the end of any functional life. By far the most debilitating of these myths was the idea that postmenopausal women had outlived their usefulness as human beings. Gail Sheehy, in *The Silent Passage,* describes menopausal and post-menopausal women as being continually upset, losing self-esteem and general performance, and ending their sexual interest and function.

Medical stereotypes, too, have traditionally defined menopause as a psychological trauma and "the trigger for a powder keg of emotions." But such inaccuracies are rapidly disappearing, thankfully. Today's researchers are disproving these stereotypes. They are discovering that most women have few, if any, psychological problems during menopause. Indeed, most women have no negative mental health consequences; in one study, only 10 percent experienced depression. In fact, normal depression is caused not by menopause, changing hormone levels, or loss of fertility, but by a reaction to financial, job, or family pressures that often coincide with menopause. Perhaps to some women, menopause seems like the last straw in a barrage of late-life challenges.

Likewise, women tend to link their emotional ups and downs to menopause. But it is the discomfort of hot flashes, which are a physical symptom of menopause, that can indirectly cause emotional distress. A woman having night sweats and losing sleep tends to feel tired, annoyed, and less able to cope. Thus, sleep deprivation, rather than a hormonal change, is the culprit.

Menopausal symptoms are often tied to expectations a woman learns from her mother. If her mother has a negative perception of menopause, she is likely to report more symptoms to her daughter. Hence, when the daughter reaches menopause, it is unclear whether her symptoms are real or the manifestation of what she has heard.

Society's attitudes can influence women's expectations, as well. While 80 percent of women in the United States report having hot flashes at least once during menopause, rarely, if ever, do Japanese women have them. Mayan women never do! In cultures that venerate elders, like certain Native American tribes and some societies in Asia, Africa, and South America, menopause is viewed as a favorable event, entitling women to new status, new privileges, and new freedom—as it ought to be.

In the West, age stereotypes give menopause a bad name, and menopausal expectations are too often realized. Amazingly, many doctors see no difference between talking about menopause and talking about aging. To link menopause with the onset of old age is utterly ridiculous. In truth, we all begin the process of aging from the day we are born.

Clearly, more study is needed. Differences between cultures may be related to environment, diet, exercise, or even fertility patterns. The Women's Health Initiative of the National Institutes of Health is tracking 100,000 middle-aged women over the next fifteen years, including Asian Americans, African Americans, Hispanics, and other groups seldom studied. This is the first longitudinal study to focus on the basics, which are reportedly "what menopause does to our bones and our skin, our sexuality and our psyche, what we go through when we go through it."

Signs and Symptoms of Menopause

Though some doctors erroneously produce a lengthy list of symptoms, only three signs can be directly attributed to the physiologic event of menopause:

1. Menstrual changes,
2. Vasomotor effect (hot flashes and night sweats), and
3. Loss of moisture and elasticity in the vagina.

Of these, no symptoms or signs are universal except for menstruation eventually stopping. In one-third of women, normal menstruation occurs right up until the periods abruptly stop. For the other two-thirds, menstrual patterns change as estrogen levels change. Periods may gradually diminish, becoming lighter or lasting fewer days, or becoming heavier and longer with ultimate cessation. Menstrual cycles may become erratic, stopping and starting with different time intervals, or simply become further and further apart.

Hot Flashes and Night Sweats

Hot flashes are the main reason women go to doctors during menopause, but the low number of women who do so suggests that most women cope on their own. The exact mechanism that causes a hot flash is unknown. We do know it is not lower estrogen levels alone, however. Women who have had low estrogen levels throughout their lives do not experience hot flashes. Evidence shows that hot flashes are initiated by the hypothalamus, the part of the brain that controls vital functions, particularly body temperature and secretion of pituitary hormones. Hot flashes could be caused by a sudden, unexplainable downward setting of the central hypothalamic thermostat.

During a hot flash, a woman's central body temperature falls. Counteractive mechanisms such as dilation of blood vessels and sweating are prompted to prevent heat loss. Blood floods into tiny blood vessels under the skin; the pulse rate rises, as does the skin temperature. Blood pressure is not affected, though. A hot flash is over in two or three minutes, but increased skin temperature and sweating may persist. Hot flashes range from being occasional and mild periods of warmth to drenching, dripping sweats accompanied by an intense feeling of heat occurring many times a day.

Some women hardly notice hot flashing:

- "I seem to have gone through menopause. It's nearly a year since I had my last period. I think I have the occasional hot flash, when I suddenly get very warm."
- "I had a hysterectomy in my early forties and had no symptoms whatsoever of menopause…not a flash, nothing…neither at the time nor later, when my ovaries went into retirement."

Hot flashes may be visible in some women as a blush or even patchy redness on the face, neck, and breasts, followed by a feeling of tiredness or chilliness. The number of women who report experiencing hot flashes is about 65 percent. Slightly

179

fewer have night sweats, which are likely a nighttime version of hot flashes.

Sex and Menopause

It is a common misconception that sexual interest and activity decline during menopause. Even doctors falsely assume that as women become older they become sexually abstinent. On the contrary, no evidence exists of a dramatic decline in desire or activity in this age group. Studies show that sex remains a vital activity for the majority of older women. When sexual activity of older women does decline, it is probably the lack of an available partner that has prompted the change, rather than a lack of interest. One study found that when women discontinued sexual relationships, only 4 percent attributed it to their own lack of interest. Researchers have shown that, while most postmenopausal women are sexually active, most who are abstinent do not have a partner, or they or their partners have medical problems.

Menopause for Thought

Let's have a "philosopause" about menopause: A fascinating phenomenon is that no other animal, not even our closest relatives—chimpanzees, monkeys, and gorillas—exhibit any evidence of menopause. All other animals remain fertile until death. Human menopause is a unique shutdown of fertility at a time when all other physiologic systems of the body continue to function. How, then, does menopause fit into Darwin's theory of evolution? What advantage, if any, does menopause offer our species?

Simply put, natural selection works to maximize the number of surviving progeny (children, in the case of humans). Why, then, does the fertility of women cease at a time in life that is barely half of total life expectancy? One explanation is that menopause is a consequence of higher survival rates in modern human societies compared to other species of animals. Menopause never occurred in the harsher circumstances in which other species evolved because death always intervened. One way of looking at it is that menopause is a measure of evolutionary success: No other species can afford to stop reproducing. On a humbler note, maybe the adaptation to cease reproduction at midlife is no great compliment to our species.

Another explanation for the evolutionary advantage of menopause lies in pre-agricultural societies, the times of hunters and gatherers. Human babies are dependent upon their mother for survival for several years after birth, and her ability to care for them declines with increasing age. In early societies, death in childbirth was common. In addition, its probability increased with the age of the mother. Probability of death for other reasons also increased with age. For instance, care of very young children was more physically demanding, increasing an older mother's risk of death. Thus, a woman's loss of fertility directly increased the probability of survival for her offspring, for when a mother enters menopause, the risk of losing her during childbirth or while caring for another child vanishes.

What You Can Do

According to Judith Bowman, senior program specialist with the American Association of Retired Persons' Women's Initiative, "The menopause experience is different for each woman; there is no right or wrong way to go through it. Some women have hot flashes, leaky bladders, or vaginal dryness; others scarcely notice any change at all. Some are sad to have lost fertility and falsely conclude they are aging more rapidly from menopause on out; others find relief from the nuisance of menstruation and the duties of child-rearing. They welcome the loss of fertility; the absence of need for contraception constitutes a distinct advantage."

There are some things you can do to help your own journey through menopause:

- Be informed. Read reliable books and articles on all aspects of menopause.
- Avoid using drugs that do not offer any physical advantage, those that seem to be manufactured mainly for profit.
- Maintain your routine. Keep active.
- Exercise. A regular exercise regimen can relieve some of the symptoms associated with menopause: hot flashes, depression, fatigue, sweating, insomnia, irritability, general muscle ache, and joint discomfort.
- Consult the most reliable doctor you can find, one who will give you the latest information about menopause and particularly the use of estrogen, progesterone, or other types of medication.

Some Final Thoughts

Research has shown what most of us already knew: Most women manage menopause in a low-key, commonsense way, not making a big deal of it. They do not regret it or regard it as a life crisis. Rather, most women are relieved not to have to worry about having their monthly periods or getting pregnant. Women's anxieties surrounding this final phase of their reproductive life are often more about aging, generally, than menopause, specifically. They are concerned about running out of the time to do all the things they want to do.

Menopause may be something of an age marker, but surely it is a positive one—a marker that announces the beginning of a new phase of life as much as it delineates the end of an old one. Menopause is a time to take account, to take risks, to slow down here, and to speed up there. One menopausal woman may have explained it best:

"About these symptoms...I suppose I'm in the midst of menopause, but I just don't pay any attention to it. I couldn't tell you at the end of the day if I've had any hot flashes or how many. It's simply one part of your entire life, why not just live it?"

Part Four

Maintaining Mental Fitness

To know how to grow old is the masterwork of wisdom,
and one of the most difficult chapters in the great art of living.
—Henri Frederic Amiel

Chapter Eleven

Don't Forget:
You Can Remember

"I must be getting old, I can't remember anything anymore."

Most people over forty voice this thought at one time or another. Memory loss is by far the most common complaint as people age. In our culture, failing memory is unfortunately as much a symbol of aging as gray hair or bifocal glasses. What most of us never learn is that most memory loss is not really lost, but has gone unused. The expectation is drilled into us that we will lose our memory as we age, and we follow the path of our expectations. As we age, there are some changes in the way our memory works, but even experts cannot agree about whether these changes are a natural part of aging or simply represent disease.

Memory can be divided into three categories: (1) immediate memory, or so-called vital memory, (2) recent memory, and (3) remote memory. Immediate memory is the ability to remember a small amount of information for a short period of time, usually seconds. The immediate memory function of older people is no different than that of younger people—that is, old people are just as capable as young people of remembering something they just heard or read.

Recent memory is the ability to learn information and retain it. The amount of information handled by recent memory is far greater than that stored in immediate memory, but it is remembered less accurately. Tests of recent memory include the ability to remember your doctor's name or several unrelated words for five to ten minutes in the presence of distraction, and the ability to learn a long sentence. An excellent test of recent memory is orientation for time and place, things that must be learned. Recent memory is thought to decline with age.

Remote memory is the ability to retrieve information learned in the past, even the distant past. Tremendous quantities of information are available to us, but we may often have difficulty remembering precise details from our childhood or other distant periods in our lives. What many are surprised to learn is that remote memory is more stable in older people than in young people. In fact, many old people focus on the past because they remember it as a time they felt better.

Scientific data supports that those who use their memory, all three types of memory, do not experience mental decline. Their memory remains as effective and functional as that of young people, some scoring even better at the ages of eighty or ninety. In truth, no one really has a poor memory, only poor learning habits or an untrained memory. Don't mistake forgetfulness, or absent-mindedness, for poor memory. More often than not, you can learn to remember.

When "known" information, a fact or date that has been stored in memory, is needed, it must be retrieved from remote memory, a slow process relative to other information processing in humans. Most of us have felt its sluggish pace when we recognize someone but can't recall his or her name. The amount of time required to retrieve information depends on the amount and intensity of exercise the memory gets. The ability to activate remote memory improves with use. Trying to remember is the mental equivalent of a physical workout. Just do it!

Old people go crazy for three reasons: (1) because of illness; (2) because they always were crazy; (3) because we drive them crazy.

—Source unknown

Treatment for Aging Brains

Many psychological tests measure speed of response. But this is a misplaced qualifier, for as we age we are less likely to guess; thus, speed should not be the only gauge. Researchers have explored whether older adults were impaired when greater processing was required, that is, if they were given a bigger load for memory to probe. The results simply depended upon the test given. For example, my mother could do a daily crossword puzzle in ten minutes, while I have never been able to complete one. Is my comparative failure the result of lack of practice or impaired processing? Certainly the former.

Why the misinformation on memory? The biggest problem is that aging itself is seen as a problem. Doctors often see what they expect to see and report only negative findings. Approximately 80 percent of people over the age of eighty-five have some cognitive memory or learning difficulties. No more than 15 percent are likely to go on to any more serious cognitive decline, however.

Dementia in old age is neither general nor common. Because patients suffering from it tend to be housed in hospitals, it is visible and frightening, but in reality, it affects only 4 to 5 percent of the sixty-five-and-older population. This is less than the percentage who go insane at earlier ages. Likewise, 9.9 per one thousand people over seventy need psychiatric hospitalization, compared with 33 per thousand in the next younger age group. This includes not only organic brain diseases, but alcoholism, depression, and ordinary insanity, as well.

189

Doctors do themselves and their patients a disservice when they diagnose memory loss as a sign of old age. It isn't. As we age, we become anxious about minor memory lapses and exaggerate the extent of the problem (if, in fact, there is a problem). Actually, the word senile is more a term of abuse than a diagnosis. It seems you're labeled senile if you make waves! But the reverse is true. Not accepting senility as a diagnosis indicates that your brain is functioning well.

When a patient complains of memory loss, doctors should take more responsibility and ask themselves whether anything they're prescribing may be causing it. In fact, numerous drugs can affect memory: digoxin, barbiturates, benzodiazepine, Valium, tricyclic antidepressants, antihistamines, diuretics, indomethacin, Naproxen, and ibuprofen. Even such commonly used drugs as septrin, compazine, Leva-dopa, bromocriptine, benzhexol, and all tranquilizers can cause confusion and compromise memory. The list is long and growing. Given this information, it is surprising that medicated elderly pass any mental tests at all!

Remember when you were six or seven and your parents noted that you had difficulty concentrating, had a short attention span, or found it difficult to learn or remember things? If you had a learning disability, you were given some special training to improve your concentration, increase your attention, or lengthen your attention span. Quite often, memory loss can also be turned around successfully. Unfortunately, the prevailing professional attitude is that old age is responsible for an inability to learn or remember. Don't let that attitude influence you.

Clinical depression (not to be confused with passing blues or the intense grief we all experience from time to time) is also a common cause of memory loss and apparent intellectual deterioration, but it is by no means permanent. Caused by the loss of concentration that typically accompanies depression, the thinking process is slowed, making it difficult to take in new information. Depression, of course, is treatable with precise doses of antidepressant drugs. Take care in selecting a qualified physician to diagnose and help you manage depression.

About 10 percent of patients who complain of impaired memory or cognition have depressive pseudodementia. Such people respond to questions with "I don't know" and frequently display emotional distress. In constrast, truly demented people respond vaguely or inappropriately.

> The true way to render age vigorous is to prolong the youth of the mind.
>
> —Mortimer Callius

What You Can Do

If you think your memory is failing, call your physician and check with your pharmacist. Ask if the medications, or combinations of medications, you are taking might alter brain functioning. To reduce the risk that brain function may be affected, your doctor may need to change dosages, substitute one drug for another, or stop them altogether. Never discontinue a prescription drug on your own, without consulting your doctor.

Physical exercise is good for you, as you know. Cerebral exercise, intellectual exertion, is just as important, even more so! Mind, as well as body, requires a workout, sort of like doing mental sit-ups or push-ups. All knowledge and memory are based on associating new information and new ideas with things you already know. The older you get, the more you know and the more you have to remember. While you have the burden of more stimuli, however, you also have the advantage of a larger base on which to connect new things, new information, and new ideas. No known limit has been found for the amount the human brain can process. With a mental fitness program, it all just happens automatically. If you haven't had what you consider a good memory in the past, I assure you, mental exercise can help you remember better than ever before.

I'll tell you a secret about my personal memory: I have a very good memory if I'm being paid for it. I'm not unusual in that regard. It seems that when money is involved everyone's memory is suddenly terrific. It's all in the motivation. If someone owed you a million dollars, you can bet you'd remember! I am driven, as are most successful people. Ego, memory, power, accomplishment, job satisfaction—money goes along with them. If you are driven, you remember what is necessary. You don't want to fail, to look foolish. And if you remember, it is obvious that you are interested.

Teaching an Old Mind New Tricks

How can you remember people, things, and locations better? Using your own experience, connect what you want to remember with anything that is funny, striking, or impressive. You need an association trigger, a reminder, to make one thing remind you of the other. How? At the moment of the action, make a silly picture (association) in your mind connecting the two vital pieces of information. The more silly, ridiculous, amusing, or impossible it is, the more likely you are to remember it and visualize instantly what you want to remember. It's the absurdity, the impossibility of the picture that takes the information out of the mundane, that makes it striking and unusual, and, therefore, easy to retrieve. Case in point: Most of us use "spring forward" and "fall back" to help us remember how to adjust our clocks.

Just making yourself attentive, paying close attention, helps dramatically. We all remember what we're interested in, so get interested in what is important to you. You remember voices on the telephone, voices heard in the hallway. Once heard and identified, they're recorded in your memory. You already have many memories of sound, automobile horns, sirens, thunder, barking dogs, meowing cats, and many more; all of these you instantly identify, even with your eyes closed.

Don't let your mind be absent. A trick I use is, if I think of something I need to do, I do it right then. Even if I'm shaving in the morning and I think of something I should write down, I stop shaving and write it down. I am sometimes criticized for this, but at least I don't forget. Another trick is to say out loud to yourself what you've just done, or what you're doing. I talk to myself a lot and that helps me remember. Common examples: "I'm unplugging the coffee pot," and "I'm locking my door."

Force yourself to think about what you're doing as you're doing it—don't allow yourself to slip into the habit of doing things automatically, without thinking. Think of the action at the moment of the action. It takes a split second to form the association, the mind picture that will work as a conscious reminder. As a wise person once said, "Thinking is the manipulation of memory. Memory failure is when you forget to think, not a poor memory."

For example, do you often search for your glasses? Connect the eyeglasses with where you're putting them by imagining a silly picture. For example, you are rushing out of the house, and on your way, you leave your glasses on a table next to a potted plant. Keep on rushing, but as you put your glasses down, visualize a pair of eyeglasses watering your potted plant with tears. Or visualize yourself wearing a potted plant over each eye instead of eyeglasses. In a split second, the image is recorded indelibly on your memory. You never stopped moving, no time was wasted—and you won't waste time searching for your glasses again. Such exaggeration helps create better and more vivid connections, which, in turn, result in stronger memories.

True memory is the associative process that is part of your genetic endowment. As you grow and mature, it's the process that makes you think white when you hear black, hot when you hear cold, in when you hear out, up when you hear down. It is the same process that opens the floodgates of memory. Recall your first-grade teacher, and you'll soon find parading into your mind the friends you had at school, fun you had on the playground, walks to and from school, and a host of other experiences that are part of you.

The associative process begins when you hear, see, or feel something with which you have been familiar in the past. You know where you were and what you were doing when John F. Kennedy was shot, only because it was such a momentous occasion, a momentous association. We are talking here about a trained memory, a mechanism enhanced by the associative capability with which you were born. The mind is an associating machine. You can easily, and often incredibly, improve what you have. The following are some tricks to train your memory:

- Learn to listen—most people don't. Think. Focus your concentration. Register information in the first place, at the moment of your awareness. Use your imagination to think up unique images to hook the new information you are hearing to your total experience. You will impress the person to whom you are listening.
- Try to remember people's names, especially when you're first introduced. Sometimes their names float over your head because you're so caught up with the social graces of trying to figure out what to say. If you didn't hear a name or were not paying attention to it, you probably won't remember it.
- Formulate retrieval cues: stop, look, listen, notice mannerisms, make observations, give whomever you meet a level gaze, eye-to-eye.
- Use the GRIP method:
    G: Get it, pay attention, ask for names to be repeated.
    R: Repeat it aloud, then repeat it to yourself; repetition makes the memory permanent.

I: Identify cues, expressions, facial expressions, face, hair, clothes, eyes.

P: Prolong memory access.

- Play games to remember things: Use imaginative images to make an association with the name. If you meet Fred Applegate, for example, visualize him as Fred Flintstone, then think of an apple sitting on a gate. The more bizarre your association, the more likely you are to remember.
- Use the rhyme technique. The name Kringer, for example, rhymes with stinger, finger, or singer. Say to yourself, "Kringer is a singer."
- Notice people's names with obvious meanings: occupations (Taylor, Baker, Carpenter, Cook, Singer, Gardener, Farmer), colors (Silver, Gray, Greene, Black, Browne, Whyte), metals or gems (Steele, Gold, Iron, Diamond, Ruby, Zircon, Opal, Pearl, Garnet), or animals (Fox, Camel, Katz, Lyons, Byrd, Swallow, Robyn, Fisch, Marlin). Even take note of names that simply remind you of something or someone: Campbell (soup), Simmonds (mattress), Carson (Johnny), Monroe (Marilyn), Carter (Jimmy), Kellogg (corn flakes), Hershey (chocolate).
- All names are potentially forgettable. (For that matter, everything is potentially forgettable.) If a name is important, review it once in a while to keep it fresh in your mind.
- Employ your mind's eye. Remember a familiar face and connect the name with it.
- Try to recall people's names twenty seconds after meeting them.
- Prepare. If you're hosting a party, review the names of your guests just before they arrive. Proper preparation prevents poor performance and memory faux pas.

- Bizarre images: Suppose you must buy gas to drive home from work. As you get out of your car, visualize something silly, such as the gas tank sitting in the seat beside you with the hose hanging out the window. You'll very likely remember to get gas.

- Parking amnesia: You go into the building where you work, and when you come out, your car doesn't seem to be there anymore. Someone moved it. The problem is, when you leave your car to go to work, you don't see the same scene as when you come back to the parking lot. So when you leave your car, stop for a moment, look back, and pay attention to what you are going to see when you return.

- Use reminders to remember things: Shift your watch to the other arm, reminding you of an appointment. Put something by the door that you need to bring along. As you get in your car and put the key in the ignition slot, say to yourself, "As I put the key in the ignition, I must remember to stop off at the shoe store and pick up my boots." Recall an introduction to someone; it may help trigger the name of the person.

- Telephone numbers or long credit card numbers: Translate it into a word. One telephone number I need to remember is the word JAKWAMO; my previous office number was KIDPETS. Or, cluster or chunk a long list of numbers; for example, telephone numbers have three sets: area code, prefix, and the suffix of the number.

- Put your rote memory to work. Long strings of associations work best, for example, fourscore and seven years. There is no limit to memory span. Rote memorization requires rehearsal—deliberate, continuous repetition of the material. Rehearsal forces the creation of a bunch of reminders and its effects last a lifetime.

- Try to remember what you just read. That is, don't read the same material three or four times and underline the important part. You're better off to read it once, then stop periodically and summarize key points.

- You are more likely to recall information if you return to the same spot where you studied it. If you're going to have a test, study in the classroom where the test will be given.
- If you can't think of a word or name, begin an alphabet search: A, B, C, D, E, F, G...this often triggers the word you are looking for. Or do a vowel search—A, E, I, O, U—to make the familiar sound.
- Maintain good health. Aerobic exercise, more oxygen pumping through your brain, helps memory.
- Do crossword puzzles.
- Do jigsaw puzzles.
- Play chess, bridge, or any card game.

Endless television commercials lure people to plastic surgery, face-lifts, body-lifts, liposuction—all presumably to look and feel younger. A "mind-lift" would sell better: Clear out, refresh, and refurbish your brain cells. Remember the common cover-up, "I can't remember your name, but your face is familiar. I never forget a face"? Rubbish! You can identify special features about any face—a wart on the nose, a wandering eye, heavy eyebrows. Use these techniques, and you will be just as good at remembering names as remembering faces.

Another good way to remember two disparate items is to merge one word to another by adding a letter, removing a letter, or changing a letter. Also, use a synonym, antonym, a word that rhymes, or any logical skip from one word to a word that the first one makes you think of. For instance: To associate key to book: key, keg, wood, paper, page, book... or key, keg, peg, pen, paper, page, book. Or, to relate book to fish, the short way: book, hook, fish. The longer way: book, look, see, sea, fish.

Next to your health, relationships with people are probably the most precious contributors to quality of life. To have any kind of relationship, you must remember things and names. You'd think this is common sense, but seemingly, it is uncommon sense, since so few people do it or even think about it.

Le Brain Jogging

Scientists in France have always had a particular interest in intellectual pursuits. They currently are using programs that exercise the brain and stimulate imagination and memory. The repertoire of this new French interest is called "le brain jogging." Techniques vary, but they all stem from the growing conviction that the more you force the brain to work as you age, the better your chances of staying alert and keeping or creating an efficient memory.

A number of different brain jogging options have developed over the past three years—namely, mechanisms of stretching, provoking, and stimulating the minds of middle-aged and older people who are eager to stay in peak form. Gerontologists in France report that these people are especially bothered by a failing memory, which specialists who are designing the system say result from anxiety, depression, and failure to demand cerebral function. The French program teaches people how memory works so they can use their own more effectively.

Le brain jogging is carried out in private clubs and clinics. Businesses and companies invite specialists to do in-house seminars. Homes and hospitals for the aged are offering training sessions. The largest and most effective of these courses was organized by a pension fund, the Mutualite Sociale Agricole, which in two years has trained counselors and started workshops in more than 120 towns and villages. Its courses consist of fifteen weekly sessions lasting two hours, and the program is called "Eureka!"

A typical Eureka session proceeds as follows: Twenty to twenty-five "joggers" between the ages of fifty-five and seventy sit around a large table and start off with a quick review of the week's news. This stimulates curiosity and initiates conversation with others. Later a psychologist projects unrelated images on a screen: a suitcase and a belt, a comb next to a fork. People are asked to remember the pairs and then establish some connection between the objects through a phrase, size, use, or material—they learn to associate. Memory is just the tip of the iceberg, though. Clients do exercises involving all mental faculties, including perception, concentration, reasoning, speech, and imagination. Of course, the problems are more or less challenging depending on the education level of the group. To learn to memorize and visualize spaces, joggers may be asked to copy a geometric design they've seen only briefly and then draw it in reverse.

Counselors usually recommend homework, which may include going shopping without a list, or memorizing a train schedule or a poem. They urge clients to play bridge, chess, and other games that require concentration and memory. Belonging to the group, counselors say, brings new confidence, new interests, and new friends. And they are doing more than reading.

> Albert Einstein fondly said, "The gift of fantasy has meant more to me than my talent for absorbing positive knowledge."

What is Learning?

All you need to know about learning anything new is that you must both understand and remember it. Simple, isn't it? Your memory is your foundation to knowledge. Few things are more satisfying than remembering something you have learned and making it a part of your total knowledge, even if it's just remembering the name of someone you met last night.

Incidentally, you may need to learn something that is quite uninteresting, even objectionable to you, in order to achieve a certain goal. Memorization occurs for no other reason than having an established habit of remembering. For example, you dial a telephone number. The line is busy. Okay, wait…count to ten…fuss and fume…try it again. Whoops, you can't remember the number. You weren't paying attention. You haven't developed the habit of paying attention to what is going on. So you have to look up the number again, or call the operator to get the number.

If memory is stored knowledge, creativity is the outcome of memory. I couldn't possibly get a million-dollar idea on how to build a better TV set; I don't know the first thing about TV sets. But I can get a creative idea on how osteoarthritis develops or even how it can be reversed, because I know about osteoarthritis. In fact, I have a massive network of bits of information in my memory about osteoarthritis. And all this information helps me find creative, individualized solutions for my patients.

I don't care how old or young you are! Above all, as you grow older, your interests (not your memory), your enthusiasm (not your memory), your endogenous drive (not your memory) may start to wane. You don't listen as attentively as you used to because you're not as interested. A large part of the solution to this is simple. Don't allow yourself to lose interest. Continue to demand your own attention. Force enthusiasm; it just needs a kick and it will light up. Make it a game. Fantasize. Sort out and work up a string of crazy ideas.

Mental exercise carries with it all the life-enhancing qualities of physical exercise. Give your brain an invigorating workout on a daily basis. It's all part of learning. Learning is the gathering of information, but there's no learning without memory. You must understand and you must remember.

For a free copy of a publication on memory by the American Association for Retired Persons, write to AARP, Fulfillment,

EE140, 1909 K Street N.W., Washington, DC 20049. Request the pamphlet "Where Did I Put My Keys?" (D13829).

Chapter Twelve

Playing the Aging Game to Win

Do you like yourself? We all have some kind of self-esteem; what varies is how positive or negative it is, or how much or little you like yourself. Just as it would be difficult for your body to stand upright without your backbone, it is difficult to handle each day emotionally without a positive self-esteem. Your self-esteem determines your ability to cope with situations, especially in later life.

Why is positive self-esteem important? It is the skeleton around which your mental health is built. People who like themselves enjoy certain characteristics: They are ready to take risks or advance in academic and vocational circles, they have more friends, they enjoy better health. Overall, they like life—they certainly live longer. People with negative self-esteem are less likely to take risks, have more trouble with performance in academic or job pursuits, have a small or diminishing circle of friends, and find it difficult to maintain relationships. They do not enjoy life nearly as much.

The most imperative psychological requirement of aging comfortably is a positive self-image: You must like yourself and be proud of who you are and your accomplishments. You must continually strive for new accomplishments and be confident that you can achieve those goals you set for yourself.

Too many of us continue to be influenced by the Puritan ethic: hard work, religious dedication, spartan lifestyle, self-reliance, and above all, humility. I grew up and was taught—in fact, it was demanded of me—to consider humility a necessary, desirable trait. But really, we should not celebrate humility. When we accomplish something we are proud of, and someone congratulates us, we tend to shuffle our feet and say, "Aw shucks, it was nothin'." Far better to say, "Yes, I was very pleased and proud."

> To be eighty years young is sometimes far more cheer-ful and hopeful than to be forty years old.
> —Oliver Wendell Holmes

Where Does Self-Esteem Come From?

What determines self-esteem? Does self-esteem determine how successful you are in life, or does life determine how positive your self-esteem is? Neither is correct all the time. Your life and your self-esteem are intimately related, certainly, but the intervening factor is how you think about it. Thus, you can improve your self-esteem simply by restructuring your cognitive techniques.

Sure, self-esteem is a great asset, but how do you acquire it? Is it a learned behavior from childhood? Self-esteem is something you have learned, and, like anything else learned, it can be changed and improved. Be your own best friend. Improve the way you feel about yourself. Every part of your life will benefit.

If you lack mental tenacity, all is not lost; it can be developed at any age. If you cope with the pressures of daily life, you are already well on your way to basic mental toughness. If you are by nature mentally strong, you probably won't have to do as much mental preparation as someone who isn't.

To begin, familiarize yourself with your negative, inappropriate thoughts. Say to yourself, "I know what you're saying, I hear you, and I'm going to stop thinking about that. I could never possibly be as bad as that!" Start with a strong, positive self-image of yourself (talk yourself into it). This may be a seminal concept to internalize at first. Not everyone feels like a winner, certainly, but even if you're 104 years old—especially if you're 104 years old—you're someone special. Believe it. Try to do a little something every day for your head.

There are several factors that work against self-esteem:

1. Society's expectations. Expectations can be inflexible. Certain behaviors are "required." But these expectations, quite simply, have nothing to do with you. It's vital to develop a coping strategy that works for you—no matter what it takes. You can learn to roll with the punches and take the ups and downs.

2. Perfectionism. Don't believe you have to be perfect. After all, who is perfect? Nobody. Are you constantly trying to achieve the impossible? If so, your self-esteem will suffer because of it. Quit being hard on yourself, and forgive yourself when you aren't perfect.

3. Criticism. Negative comments by others hit home more deeply than they should. Working on your thinking is the first step in dealing with criticism. Recognize everyone's right to criticize, but also recognize the positive messages behind critical comments.

4. Passivity. Elderly people tend to be passive, letting others go before them, counting others' feelings and opinions as more important than their own. You can learn assertiveness. "Pulling rank" is one of the rights and pleasures of age—think of it as an entitlement. Courteously but firmly, show people you value yourself and expect them to value you. Be ruthless toward rudeness or brush-offs, if necessary. If you have a disability, it's wise to make others, such as flight attendants, bus drivers, or salespeople, aware of it. If you were a well-known V.I.P. they'd offer special treatment; you're entitled as a privilege of your age.

Along the same lines, ask for help when you need it. Cash in on the kindness and generosity you gave earlier in life. People often fear that elderly people will see an offer to help as an infringement on their independence. If you need help, it's your right to ask for it, not an imposition. You may be surprised at how nicely people go along with the idea that you merit respect. You just have to show that you expect it.

> There is beauty in extreme old age.
> Do you fancy you are elderly enough,
> Information I'm requesting
> On a subject interesting
> Is a maiden all the better when she's tough?
> —W. S. Gilbert, *The Mikado*

Imagery and Visualization

I purposely put the psychological aspects of aging at the end of the book because I firmly believe that a positive mental approach is the most essential ingredient in winning the aging game. The most influential and basic psychological requirement for success is self-image. You achieve it by visualizing yourself performing at a high level, successfully competing in the aging game, even though you are only competing against yourself. Visualize not how you think you are, but how you want to be. Visualization is every bit as important as physical conditioning, and it is like physical conditioning in that the more you do it, the better you get at it.

Positive visualization, or mental imagery, is viewing yourself as successful, unveiling a strong, positive self-image, which results in confidence and self-worth. The subconscious mind doesn't know the difference between reality and what you imagine. Thus, what you visualize is going to happen can, in fact, happen. Establish in your mind an attitude of quiet confidence. Picture yourself achieving your goal and imagine having already accomplished it.

Scientific studies confirm how effective imagery is. One study used a randomly selected group of basketball players who were tested on their ability to shoot basketball foul shots. Each player was asked to attempt a number of shots, and a percentage score based upon successful shots was recorded. Then three groups were formed, each having an identical cumulative score from the first test. Group 1 was told to avoid any basketball practice or foul shot shooting for one month. Group 2 practiced shooting foul shots an hour a day during the month. Group 3 was instructed not to touch a basketball for the month, but to visualize successfully shooting foul shots for one hour each day.

When the groups rejoined one month later, researchers were not surprised by the results of Groups 1 and 2: Group 1 made no improvement in total score, and Group 2 significantly improved. But the results of Group 3 blew their minds. Though they had not touched a basketball during the month, Group 3 members improved only slightly less than Group 2, and far more than Group 1.

Imagery works, and it works best when it is realistic. Use all your senses: sight, hearing, smell, taste, touch, as well as the proprioceptive sense, which tells you where all your body parts are. Make your visualization as complete as possible. See yourself accomplishing your task, but incorporate the whole scene. See the foreground and background, hear surrounding noises, smell the smells, taste the tastes, feel the power of your muscles. Experience the sense of balance in your body, its efficiency. Eliminate all distractions that distract you from your goal. Positive imagery works at any age, but you do have to practice visualization and develop a technique that is right for you.

The messages you send your subconscious are critical to your self-image. Suppose you plan to go sailing in the morning but find when you get up that it is raining hard and there is little wind. This is an opportunity to make a situation positive. As they say, "When life gives you lemons, make lemonade." Think of an indoor activity that's fun and interesting, one you've been meaning to do for awhile: phoning friends or relatives, renting a movie, catching up with letters, or writing in your journal. Or, if your self-esteem is already high and in need of a challenge, go sailing anyway and pit yourself against the elements. Life has always been a series of daily victories and defeats. Bucking the negative side is of great importance.

Improving self-esteem through visualization doesn't just happen; it is a talent developed, like any other talent. Celebrate aging. Test your mental toughness. Tell yourself: "Right now there's nothing I'd rather be doing than playing the aging game. I am who and where I want to be."

He that has seen both sides of fifty, has lived to little purpose if he has not other views of the world than he had when he was much younger.

—William Cowper

Loneliness

We tend to think of old age as a lonely time. We see the images on TV of old people "warehoused" in institutions, unattended, bored, abandoned. Sometimes, this is the case. Some people do complain about feeling abandoned in their golden years. But for the majority of the elderly, these images couldn't be further from the truth. Of course, being alone is totally different from feeling lonely. Being alone can be a satisfying choice. I like being alone: There's nobody I know better, and who else can I really trust?

Loneliness is being alone when you don't want to be. As evidenced by the statistics on suicide, the elderly are not alone in their loneliness. Cities contain lonely people of all ages. It's quite unlikely that loneliness is any more common in later life than in early and middle life. But as we age, two factors do increase our chances for loneliness: bereavement and illness.

After years of living with a loved one, it's especially difficult to get over it when that person dies—even more difficult than it might have been earlier in life. Of women in America, 70 percent can expect to be widowed. Yet most do not consider how they will handle it when it happens. Perhaps it is too great a chore to get over the loss of a spouse. As someone once sensitively expressed it for tens of thousands, "It's hardly worth going home."

Illness also increases the chance for loneliness in old age. Many people who become ill, psychologically or physically or both, lose mobility and gradually reduce their involvement in life. They slowly lose their contacts and friendships. Sadly, many become bitter because of the "treatment" they've received in life, from society in general, but most often from themselves. In fact, they may make themselves ill or unpleasant to be around.

Society's stereotypes of aging do not help, either. Outlets like work are healing for people in mourning, but age discrimination often prevents seniors from working. A great dam of unhappiness could be set free if older people were expected to work and allowed to do so. Work, unless it's completely solitary, is a superb antidote to loneliness. Likewise, groups such as Senior Citizens Centers can help. But shop for a good one, with more than bingo and shuffleboard. Fitness, nutrition, mental gymnastics, and craft classes are far more productive. Community organizations that promote the elderly's rights are even better.

I hope for an ideal: a people center, without meaningless age limits. Still, it has to start somewhere. We might combine communal dining with educational and activist training, an employment organization, and an advice-to-lovers bureau. And for the few people who don't, won't, or cannot go out, I envision a volunteer arm of this people center, who seek out the elderly holed up in their homes and visit them. Meals on Wheels is one such program and could be used as a template.

Some people simply will not accept help, and this is the case among all age groups. The majority, however, welcome such attention. Some so-called shut-ins may have stairs they are afraid to climb or descend. They may need to regain their sense of self, their personhood. The turnaround produced by vigorous community concern is often amazing.

Of course, we wouldn't be so amazed if we thought about it and felt more kinship with the elderly. If you're lonely but can walk, get such an operation going. Even if it's just for one person at first, you may still find that, in the process of helping another, you cure your own loneliness.

How about the word love? It is multipurpose, certainly. I love my spouse, my children, my country, my parents, hard rock music, the oldies, the golden oldies, horses, skiing, running, all in different ways. Still, the most common interpretation of love is sexual; only secondarily is love considered lifelong.

Love is what preserves us. Love is ideal if the object is a person, but also valuable is a love of music, literature, a special place, job, pet, and so forth. A person at eighty who can love, in any sense of the word, is a person who has maintained contact with something or somebody.

Developing love takes time and effort, and enables you to relish your own as well as others' capacity to love. We often neglect the elderly, and in the process exclude them from the normal daily social experiences. This profoundly damages them. In fact, isolation is a common cause of senility. Aging interferes with sensory avenues. Sight is dimmed, hearing and proprioception are reduced. Diminishing flexibility discourages the search for sights and sounds. This form of isolation, which is completely unnecessary, results in impaired thinking, altered emotional response, disturbed visual function, hallucination, and changes in brain wave patterns. Variety is not just the spice of life—it is the very stuff of it.

The art of living consists of dying young—but as late as possible. —Anonymous

---

Goals

As we age, we tend to set fewer goals, assuming it's all downhill from here. This is wrong for playing the aging game to win. Clear goals serve a crucial function: They initiate and demand decisions, consciously and subconsciously. Hitch your wagon to a star—make the sky the limit! We would have never gotten to the moon without setting goals. Always have goals, multiple goals, that are appropriate and possible, but not too easy to attain. It's best to avoid goals that involve other people, since you want to influence your own performance. Sometimes setting a series of progressive goals works well.

We tend to be too realistic in life. Why not begin now to think what is possible, not just what is probable? Plan to set some records, and break some others. Records are made to be broken, and if broken, it won't be by much. Record—the very word sets my juices flowing.

English novelist and critic John Cowper Powys had the superior, privileged education of upper-class Britain. He was acutely knowledgeable about the foundations of Western civilization, and was able to write with authority on all aspects of its society, political, social, or literary. Yet he later realized he had studied philosophy, not learning; he had learned beliefs, not knowledge. At age sixty, he set out to reach some

211

perception of order about the world. He wrote in his autobiography, "My life's about to begin." From that point on, his life became a search for meaning. He lived to be ninety-one. Talk about setting new goals!

> Grow old along with me!
> The best is yet to be,
> The last of life, for which the first was made.
> —Robert Browning, "Rabbi Ben Ezra"

Time

Managing time efficiently is as vital in the later years as it is during the peak of a career. Your time is as valuable now as ever. The only way to gain or save time is to spend it wisely and effectively; age has nothing to do with it.

Forgetting is still one of the biggest infringements on effective time management. Don't put off something that needs to be done now. Don't let any piece of paper, order, or plan go through your hands more than once. Just do it. This million-dollar idea is the essence of many time management seminars, but actually it is more a memory aid than anything else. If you do it as soon as you think of it, it's impossible to forget. If you don't, a month later it turns up and it's another head-banging moment: "Damn it, I forgot about this!"

Watch a short-order cook sometime. No matter what order is called out, the cook instantly takes out one key ingredient to remind him or her of the order. A strip of bacon on the grill is better than a string around the finger. A string only reminds people that they wanted to remember something. The strip of bacon is part of that something to remember, and is followed by more bacon, lettuce, tomato, and bread.

Forcing recollection with the obvious is called linking. Make a link that tells you what you're going to do today. Forming a link will make you remember things you plan to do, force you to plan your day, and reinforce your commitment to effective time management.

Sports Psychology

I am a student of, and entranced by the whole area of sports psychology. Mental training for sports borders on magic: Alterations in thought and perception inspire physical feats that almost defy logic, and certainly defy prediction. Are physical activity, self-esteem, daily performance, productivity, optimism, and health related? I think so. As you age, can you master mental education and training as well as younger people do? Can we condition aging minds as well as bodies? Does competitiveness have to diminish or disappear with increasing age? Is it necessary for people over fifty to suffer psychological burnout and depression, looking forward only to their exit from this life and remaining on a downhill slide until it occurs?

In some ways, the way athletes prepare psychologically for competition is pertinent to the aging game. I look on the aging game as a sport to be approached with all the curiosity, anticipation, and eagerness that characterized earlier parts of my life, only without the uncertainties and delusions of those years.

Only recently has mental training received as much attention as physical training. Human thought is a complex, sophisticated, amazing, and continuous process. Its role in regaining and maintaining overall health is a vital one, and should be used in later years. Athletes at all ages arouse themselves emotionally to perform as required. They do this with self-talk, muscle relaxation, deep breathing, and other techniques. Similar to visualization and imaging, this type of mental control can actually improve physical skills. Among marathon runners, for instance, 85 to 90 percent of their performance is based on how strong they are mentally on the day of the race.

If sports psychology is so powerful a factor in physical ability and performance, why hasn't it become available to aging people? Mostly, because it is still relatively new. Sports psychology is a profession still struggling with identity and development. Great progress has been made, but far greater progress will surely be made in the next few decades. In the meantime, however, we can use the available techniques and attitudes to play the aging game to win.

Years ago, the United States biathlon ski team hired Marie Alkire as a rifle coach. She was a national champion, and a product of the famous advanced marksmanship training center at Fort Benning, Georgia. Her most lasting contribution to the team was a manual she wrote on mental training. The opening sentence reads, "Shooting is 90 percent mental, once the technical skills have been mastered."

> When I was young I was amazed at Plutarch's statement that the elder Cato began at the age of 80, to learn Greek. I am amazed no longer. Old age is ready to undertake tasks that youth shirked because they would take too long.
>
> —William Somerset Maugham

Self-Talk

The first step in mental control is to start listening to yourself. Most of us spend great amounts of time in unrecognized thought, chattering away without focusing on or listening to ourselves. This type of internal self-talk occurs any time we're not speaking. Tune in to your stream of consciousness. Begin by identifying situations when you are usually silent and thinking:

daydreaming, driving a car, exercising, taking a shower. Then, tune in. At first, you'll need to remind yourself to do this. The more you listen to yourself, the more automatic it will be.

The next step is learning to identify negative self-talk. For example, if you find yourself thinking you're tired, yet no physical symptoms of fatigue are present, why are you telling yourself you are tired? Maybe you are bored, or feel lazy at that point. Thinking you are tired is tiring. Instead, think about something else, something positive. Control your mind; don't allow self-defeating, critical, upsetting thoughts.

As we age, we tend to engage in negative self-talk more often. We self-blame, even verbally self-abuse, if we fail at anything, including our unrealistic goals. It is easier to imagine that we're going downhill, that we'll always be less than we were in our youth. We begin to imagine things that can go wrong or block our success. Don't be guilty of this negative attitude. Too often, negativity creeps in and, like the weather, we accept it, convinced we can do nothing about it. We can, though.

Send a positive message to your subconscious. It is critically important to your self-image. Even if you can't change your environment, you can still change your perception of it. Surround yourself with positive people and absorb their mood. Create a positive attitude and plan: "I'm as good as anybody here—I'm eighty, I'm experienced, and I know about life." Soon, you'll find that by creating a positive self-image, those around you will have a positive image of you.

I talk to myself all the time. I'm not lying to myself, but rather asking my head to be creative. I'm being optimistic by my own volition. To see things in a positive light, call on your talent and experience. Be kind to yourself. Praise yourself. Be tolerant when you don't live up to your expectations. Show yourself, or find a way to learn, how to achieve whatever you want to accomplish. Talk yourself into believing who you are. Pathologic optimism is not a bad way to be.

Young men think old men are fools; but old men know young men are fools.

—George Chapman

Arousal and Relaxation

In sports psychology, the optimal range of arousal is narrow. When you have not reached the proper level, you will not perform at your best. But when you become overly aroused, to the point of feeling nervous, your performance will suffer, too.

How can you tell if you are psyched up or psyched out? Gauging your mental arousal, to say the least, is elusive. It is difficult to isolate, let alone evaluate. For this reason, coaches tend to concentrate on physical performance, the logic being that if an athlete is doing everything right, he or she needs no coach. This type of coaching is becoming obsolete as the sports world learns the value of mental training, however. Most of us are familiar with the importance of physical warmups for improving athletic performance, but few of us realize that a psychological warmup is just as important for optimum mental performance.

A single deep breath, fully controlled, immediately reduces the heart rate. Thus, a combination of calming self-talk and relaxation can reduce the state of arousal. If you are anxious in large crowds, for example, you might take a deep breath and say to yourself, "I'm not comfortable here with all these spectators, but I can handle it." Then, as you slowly exhale, tell yourself to relax as you let the tension drain from your body.

Relaxation is as essential as arousal. For champion athletes, who are frequently overachievers, the relaxation response becomes a talent they must acquire and use daily. Relaxation response has always been a component of religious teachings. Its use is most widespread in Eastern cultures, where it is an essential part of everyday existence. The physiology of relaxation response has only recently been researched, defined, and reproduced in the West.

> No wise man ever wished to be younger.
> —Jonathan Swift

Relaxation Exercise

Relaxation response is actually quite simple. It requires four elements:

1. A quiet environment.

2. A mental device, such as a word or phrase—this is repeated in a specific fashion over and over again, a mantra. The word *one* is often used. I use *orioles*, because I like the liquid sound of r's and l's.

3. The absence of thought—a blank, clear, passive attitude is probably the most important of these four elements.

4. A comfortable position, sitting or lying down.

The following is the narrative of a relaxation exercise. It can be recorded, so you can guide yourself by listening to your tape, or you can mentally guide yourself through a relaxation exercise.

Get as comfortable as you can. Uncross your arms and legs. Have nothing on your lap. Loosen tight clothing or jewelry. Close your eyes.

Slowly breathe in through your nose and blow out through your mouth. Completely fill your lungs with air and breathe out slowly. Breathe in again slowly, deeply, at your own relaxed pace. Breathe from your diaphragm. Focus all your attention on your breathing.

Repeat [your word] after each breath. Do not concentrate on any thoughts that come into your mind. Don't fight or resist them, just concentrate on your breathing and [the word you are repeating]. Imagine you are breathing in relaxation and breathing out tension, so that with each breath, you are more and more relaxed.

Let your body breathe, according to its own natural rhythm; slowly, deeply. Let go of any remaining tension in your body; let the tension melt away. Continue to breathe in relaxation and breathe out tension. With each breath, you feel more and more relaxed.

Whenever you're ready, slowly open your eyes and stretch. Practice this exercise for fifteen to twenty minutes once a day, up to as many as four times a day. At the end of each session, you will feel not only relaxed and comfortable, but also energized. You will find such a powerful sense of well-being that you will easily be able to meet any demands that arise.

All Work and No Play

Play is not just for children. Random play, with no particular goal, is the best way to get our minds to turn up what we want to know. Play is a way to tap the unconscious, to lay bare and connect hidden ideas and knowledge. All of us engaged in the aging game need to play. Play is a problem solver. Interpretation and revelation occurs while the mind is at play. When the mind is not under pressure, it works with a certain automaticity. The play of the body, mind, and spirit is its own reason for being. In its purposelessness, it achieves a purpose.

The discovery experience—psychologists call it the Aha! phenomenon—is a sudden insight, a flash of inspiration, or the discovery of a long-sought solution. The mind effortlessly takes information, repositions it, fusses around with ideas, and finds unrecognized associations. I find that letting my mind idle while I walk allows mental mechanisms to either solve problems or turn up some idea, concept, or revelation. Chances are, these insights would not have come to me unless I let my mind play.

Exercise Deficiency

Are you feeling run down? Tired by two in the afternoon? Is getting to work too much for you? Are you depressed? Do you lack initiative? Are you tired most of the time? The "ailment" from which you are most likely suffering is exercise deficiency. Exercise deficiency is a disease of lifestyle that affects about half the people in the United States. In my opinion, it is the most prevalent cause of sickness in America.

Full-blown exercise deficiency is easy to identify: Any activity is an effort. Repose is your natural state. You are fatigued early in the day. Most people with exercise deficiency are unaware they've "caught" it. They believe their lack of energy and initiative is part of the aging process. They think they are normal.

They aren't. Slowing down, becoming less productive, experiencing a decrease in physical work capacity—that's average, but it's not normal. Ebbing of life can occur at any age. But such attitude-induced loss of physical and intellectual capability usually strikes people in their mid-thirties and worsens with age. This sort of thinking has caused the epidemic of exercise deficiency in the United States. To be functional, optimistic, and have a positive self-image, you must be physically fit, whether you're twenty-five, forty-five, one hundred, or older.

Hippocrates (460-377 B.C.) said it best: "That which is used develops, and that which is not used wastes away." Fatigue, exhaustion, decline in productivity—these are direct results of diminishing levels of fitness. Heart, lung, joint, or kidney diseases, too, are caused by a simple case of severe exercise deficiency. The good news is, the effects of exercise deficiency are reversible at any age by beginning an exercise program.

People with these diseases tend to become blind to the value of exercise. But a patient with extensive kidney disease can still exercise. It won't cure his or her kidneys, of course, but kidneys are not the cause of a sedentary, restricted, and

219

compromised existence. Exercise deficiency is a self-inflicted disease. It's all around us. Take responsibility for getting the most out of your own body and your life, whatever the limitations.

Aerobic Exercise after Fifty

Some of us over age fifty have a secret: Our energy levels are higher than ever before and we exude a new sense of optimism and vigor that the young don't have. How? After the age of fifty, regular aerobic exercise induces innumerable changes in the body and mind, the aggregate of which is called the training effect.

The human body is designed to adapt to aerobic exercise by delivering oxygen from the lungs to the muscles. This is accomplished by changes in blood circulation, the brain, the heart, and the lungs. Blood volume increases and the amount of oxygen-carrying hemoglobin in red blood cells increases. The heart is able to move larger amounts of blood with each beat, decreasing the number of heartbeats needed to circulate the blood. Muscles involved in exercise inherently have a greater capacity to use oxygen. When oxygen is present, energy is produced in tiny inclusions called mitochondria, the power-houses of the cells. With continued exercise, these packets (mitochondria) increase in both number and size. So as the delivery of oxygen is improved and more oxygen is delivered, more energy is produced. The result: You can do more, both physically and mentally.

With regular exercise, lung capacity increases, oxygen is moved more rapidly to the blood, and the ability to breathe more air per minute rises. Ligaments, tendons, bone, cartilage, and capsules of joints develop increased tensile strength as well as compressive strength. Although these changes occur more slowly than those in the heart and lungs, they can occur at any age—at ninety, or even one hundred twenty!

Research suggests that the improvements in attitude, mental outlook, and self-image that result from regular exercise reduce tension and anxiety, and increase self-discipline, motivation, and self-determination. Of course, following an exercise regimen faithfully requires a balance of inspiration and discipline. But a funny thing happened on the way to your golden years. An internal discipline developed that allows you to accomplish much more than you could in your twenties, thirties, or forties. You now have something that can't be bought. The only way to get it is to live it. That something is experience.

It is not an easy task to age gracefully. Aging gracefully means aging happily and healthfully. Accept who you are. Trade off a state of becoming for a state of being. That's what aging is. You've arrived. Why not continue being your best until the final buzzer?